NUTRITION FOR THE HEALTH PROVIDER

Self-Care and Patient Guidance

NUTRITION FOR THE HEALTH PROVIDER

Self-Care and Patient Guidance

by

Vanessa Baute, MD

Jessica Deffler, MD

Wake Forest University School of Medicine

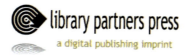

ISBN 978-1618460325

First Printing

Copyright © 2017 by the Authors

All images reproduced with permission.

All rights reserved,
including the right of reproduction,
in whole or in part, in any form.

Produced and Distributed By:

Library Partners Press
ZSR Library
Wake Forest University
1834 Wake Forest Road
Winston-Salem, North Carolina 27106

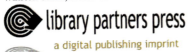

www.librarypartnerspress.org

Manufactured in the United States of America

The authors

dedicate this book to

farmers

and to all those dedicated to

the cause of sustainable nutrition.

ACKNOWLEDGMENTS

The authors would like to thank:

- The Student Wellness Department at Wake Forest University for funding the publication of this book for their medical students;
- The Center for Integrative Medicine at Wake Forest Baptist Health for their support and encouragement of this project;
- The Arizona Center for Integrative Medicine for paving the way for physicians to receive training in holistic care of patients including nutrition education;
- Our families for listening to us talk about food ad nauseum; and,
- Library Partners Press for delicious expertise and creativity.

Together we seek to bring nutrition into the curriculum of more medical schools around the country and globe.

SPECIAL THANKS

And special thanks to *Pamela Rosado* for the original photography, and for her passion for good food.

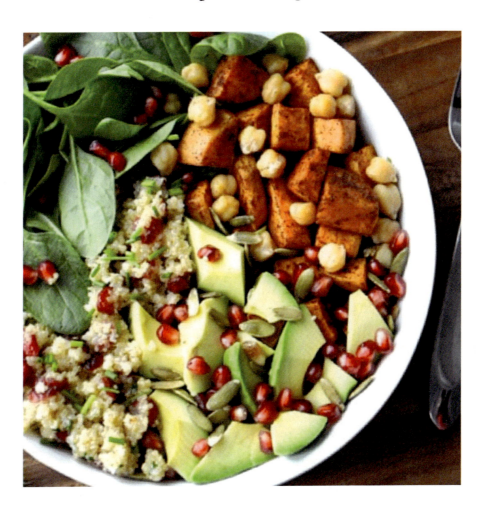

ABOUT THE AUTHORS

Vanessa Baute, MD received her neurology training at the Medical College of Georgia. She studied the role of food as medicine during her Integrative Medicine fellowship at the University of Arizona. Dr. Baute currently practices as an integrative neurologist, assistant professor and director of Integrative Medicine education at Wake Forest Baptist Medical Center.

Jessica Deffler, MD completed her medical education at Wake Forest School of Medicine and is pursuing a residency in Family Medicine at Thomas Jefferson University Hospital in Philadelphia, PA. She looks forward to incorporating nutrition into her practice and is especially interested in access to healthy food for the underserved.

CONTENTS

PART ONE: OVERVIEW, 1

    Nutrition Basics
        Whole-foods versus processed foods
        Plant-based nutrition
        What's in your food?
        Fiber
        Fats
        Carbohydrates
        Protein
    Cooking at home
        Plant-based kitchen staples
        Food comparison
        Healthy meal swaps
    Healthy on a Budget
        Organic food

PART TWO: HEALTHY EATING, 33

    Special sections
        The anti-inflammatory diet
        Vitamins
    Patient Guidance
    Motivational interviewing

PART THREE: DIET AND DISEASE, 45

    Evidence-Based Nutrition as Medicine
    Obesity
    Intuitive Eating
    Diabetes
    Cardiovascular
    Hypertension
    Cancer
    Antioxidants
    Gastrointestinal disease
    Neurologic disease
    Headache
    Cognitive Impairment

PART FOUR: RECIPES, 77

    Breakfast
    Lunch
    Dinner
    Dessert

REFERENCES, 103

PART ONE: OVERVIEW

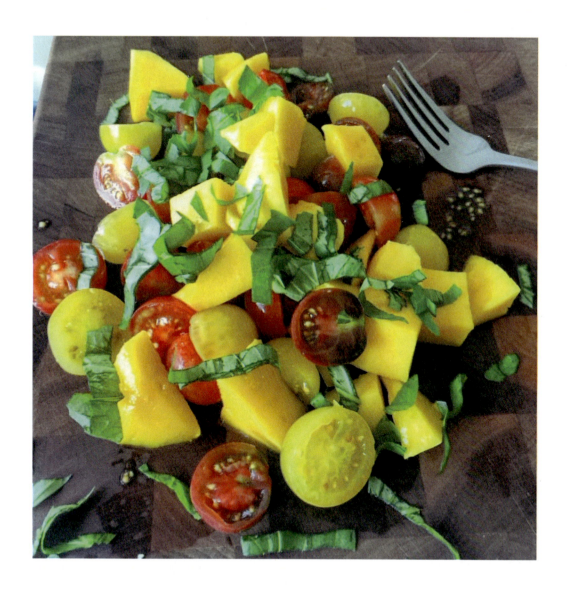

INTRODUCTION: WHY IS THIS IMPORTANT?

> *We need to focus on overall nutrition quality. We need to be more pragmatic, and less dogmatic. And we need guidance that extends to the full range of food choices people actually make every day."*
> —David Katz, MD, *"Living [and Dying] on a Diet of Unintended Consequences"*

Attempting to change our own diets and make recommendations to patients can be overwhelming. Fad diets are abundant, and patients may have tried low-carb, low-fat, high-protein, or "detox" diets. They may have questions about vitamins, supplements, fiber, fried food, organic food and more.

Perhaps we can simplify it all. What we need is to emphasize *overall* quality of what we eat. We already know what foods can promote health and prevent chronic disease, and there is literature to support it. A whole-food, plant-based diet, rich in vegetables, fruits, whole grains, healthy fats, and plant-based protein provides optimal nutrition and prevents disease.[1] Healthy eating does not over-restrict or over-emphasize a particular food group, but rather encourages healthful food choices within those groups. It encourages us to return to a diet that more closely resembles that of our ancestors and traditional cultures, and to reject the mass-consumer, large-portion, processed food that is making ourselves and our patients sick. Overall, changing the state of nutrition in America will require large-scale changes in culture and food access. Physicians cannot solve the problem alone, but we will be vital to the change toward a healthy eating America. We can start by educating ourselves.

This nutrition guide emphasizes the importance of food, including its role in preventing and treating chronic disease. The goal is to educate ourselves as future physicians and to use our personal experience with food to guide our patients in their individual nutrition journeys.

NUTRITION BASICS

PROCESSED FOODS VERSUS WHOLE FOODS

Americans live in a culture of processed food, the focus of which is profit – not the source of ingredients or the health impact on the eater. Processed food is manufactured to cause addiction, leaving the eater with an insatiable feeling. *For example, compare natural versus processed sugar – have you ever found it difficult to stop eating bananas? Probably not. Now what about cookies?*

◊ Processed foods, high calorie snacks, and sugary beverages are readily available and cheap.

◊ Fast food is tasty, high in saturated fats and trans-fats, processed meat, and refined carbs and sugar. It is served in large portions and often with sugary drinks.

◊ Processed foods contain additives and artificial ingredients, for example monosodium glutamate and hydrogenated oils, which contribute to their addictive effect. Even ingredients listed as "natural flavors" are artificial and inhibit satiety.

◊ The most addictive foods appear to be those that are highly processed and high in fat and glycemic load (for example, fast food, pizza, and chocolate).[2]

◊ A few studies have looked at dopamine activity in the brain to describe food addiction.[3] Dopamine is the neurotransmitter involved in reward and addiction. A study using PET scans showed decreased dopamine sensitivity in the brains of obese individuals, similar to the patterns seen in those with cocaine addiction.

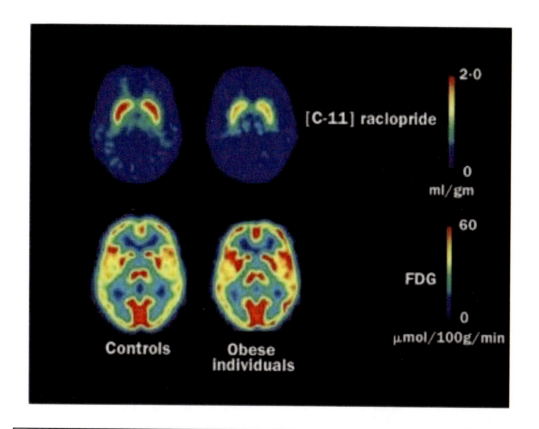

Positive Emission Tomography (PET) scans of dopamine uptake in normal (left) and obese (right) subjects, demonstrating reduced dopamine sensitivity in patients whose diets contained large amounts of fast food.[4]

In contrast to processed and fast food, whole foods are processed as little as possible and contain no artificial ingredients or additives. They contain the most health benefit. In fact, many studies support the concept of whole foods as medicine.

PLANT-BASED NUTRITION

Eat food. Not too much. Mostly plants.
– Michael Pollen, In Defense of Food: An Eater's Manifesto

Data from the CDC shows that **<18% of adults consume the recommended daily intake of fruit (1.5-2 cups) and <14% consume the daily recommended intake of vegetables** (2-3 cups).[5]

The majority of chronic disease is preventable with a whole-food, plant-based diet. As a powerful example, a 2014 cohort study by Dr. Caldwell Esselstyn and others showed that a vegan, plant-rich diet is capable of reversing coronary artery disease.[6]

Tenants of plant-based, whole-food nutrition include

- Eat mostly plants – vegetables, whole fruits, legumes, and whole grains.
- Eat mostly "energy dilute foods" – foods that cause satiety with fewer calories, due to their higher water and fiber content.
- Eat mostly plant-based sources of protein, such as lentils, quinoa, beans, nuts and seeds.
- Incorporate healthy (monounsaturated and polyunsaturated) fats.
- Avoid foods that come in a box; these tend to be processed and costly.
- Limit or eliminate fast food and sugar-sweetened beverages.
- Reconnect with food through cooking, and consider buying local produce.

Does plant-based mean vegetarian/vegan?

Not necessarily - it means switching proportions to make plants the majority of the plate, substituting high-quality meat sparingly.

◊ Vegetarianism and veganism are associated with longer lifespan and lower incidence of diabetes, heart disease, and cancer.[7]
◊ The benefits of a vegetarian diet come from the higher consumption of vegetables (especially leafy greens) and fruits, whole grains, and plant-based protein, as well as the avoidance of red and processed meat.
◊ A vegetarian diet naturally contains less unhealthy fat and more fiber.
◊ All meat is not created equal. The processed meat of today is different from that which our ancestors consumed. In addition, grass-fed beef, which is fed the natural diet of the cow, is not the same as factory-farmed beef, which is fed synthetic grains and antibiotics.
◊ A vegetarian/vegan diet is also better for the environment (which in turn affects our health). The beef and milk industries contribute significantly to greenhouse gas emissions.[9] In addition, one-third of all farmable land is used for livestock and poultry.

Did you know?
More than half of all antibiotic use in the US is by the meat production industry, used to make animals grow larger and avoid disease in crowded and unsanitary conditions.[8]

Bottom line – Vegetarian or not, eat a generous variety of fruits and vegetables. Limit processed and red meat. If you like fish, eat wild salmon at least twice weekly (or supplement with a high quality fish oil supplement.)

WHAT'S IN YOUR FOOD?

In this section, we will take a closer look at the nutrients in food –

- ◊ Fiber
- ◊ Fats
- ◊ Carbohydrates
- ◊ Protein

> Reading food labels helps us to find healthy nutrients and avoid unhealthy additives.

Nutrition Facts	
Serving size: 1/4 cup	
Amount per serving	
Calories 170 Cal from Fat 120	
% Daily Value	
Total Fat 13g	20%
Saturated Fat 2.5g	12%
Trans Fat 0g	
Cholesterol 0mg	0%
Sodium 10mg	0%
Total Carbohydrate 4g	1%
Dietary Fiber 2g	8%
Sugar 2g	
Protein 8g	
Vitamin content	

Peanuts
High in fat but full of protein

Nutrition Facts	
Serving size: 1 container (150g)	
Amount per serving	
Calories 110 Cal from Fat 0	
% Daily Value	
Total Fat 0g	0%
Saturated Fat 0g	0%
Trans Fat 0g	
Cholesterol 0mg	0%
Sodium 65mg	2%
Total Carbohydrate 15g	5%
Dietary Fiber 0.5g	2%
Sugar 12g	
Protein 12g	24%
Vitamin content	

Peach Greek yogurt, 0%
Non-fat but with added sugar

Nutrition Facts	
Serving size: 1 package	
Amount per serving	
Calories 150 Cal from Fat 70	
% Daily Value	
Total Fat 8g	12%
Saturated Fat 1.5g	7%
Trans Fat 0g	
Cholesterol 0mg	0%
Sodium 180mg	7%
Total Carbohydrate 17g	6%
Dietary Fiber 1g	6%
Sugar 1g	
Protein 2g	
Vitamin content	
Ingredients: Corn, vegetable oil, whey, monosodium glutamate, buttermilk, romano cheese, whey protein concentrate, etc.	

Doritos
High in fat and empty of nutrients

THE BENEFITS OF FIBER: BEYOND THE BATHROOM

Fiber is carbohydrate from plants that is indigestible and passes through the intestines largely unchanged. Most Americans eat between 15 and 20 grams of fiber daily.[10] **Our Paleolithic ancestors consumed 100g daily!**[11] Facts on fiber –

- ◊ There is no fiber in meat and dairy.
- ◊ Refined grains (including white bread, white and enriched flour, and crackers) have been processed, removing most of the fiber.
- ◊ Recommended fiber intake is **22-28g** (women) **and 28-34g** (men).
- ◊ Fiber's satiating effect aids weight loss and helps prevent obesity.
- ◊ High fiber intake reduces cholesterol and blood pressure.
- ◊ Fiber reduces risk of constipation, diverticulosis, hemorrhoids, and possibly colon cancer.

Fiber – Bottom Line

- ◊ Eat a variety of legumes, vegetables, and fruits.
- ◊ Switch from white rice (less than 1g of fiber per cup) to whole grains such as quinoa.
- ◊ Try **whole wheat pasta (6g fiber per cup)** instead of white pasta (2g fiber).
- ◊ Check the whole grains label for **at least 16g per serving**.
- ◊ Bread is not a whole grain, but if eating it, aim for at least 2g fiber per slice.
- ◊ Fruit skins contain fiber and the antioxidant quercetin.[12] Try whole fruit or smoothies instead of juicing.

GOOD FATS, BAD FATS

Not all fats are unhealthy; it's the *quality* and the portion of fats that matters. For example, the traditional Mediterranean diet is relatively high in total fat from olive oil, nuts, and seeds, but is associated with lower risk of heart disease and diabetes.[1] The difference is that it emphasizes healthy fats in healthy portion sizes.

◊ **Polyunsaturated and monounsaturated fats** are derived from plant-based sources – plant oils (olive oil, canola oil), nuts (especially walnuts), black olives, and avocados.

◊ Monounsaturated fatty acid (MUFA) and polyunsaturated fatty acid (PUFA) intake is associated with decreased mortality.

◊ A recent review showed that replacing 5% of calories from saturated fat with an equivalent amount from PUFAs was associated with 27% reduction in mortality.[13]

◊ **Trans-fat** is found in processed food and fast food, and intake has been associated with atherosclerosis and increased mortality.

◊ **Saturated fat** is associated with obesity and increased mortality, but source matters.
    o Healthier sources (in moderation) include coconut oil, dark chocolate, and nuts.
    o Unhealthy sources include red/processed meat and the cooking oils used in fast food.
    o Butter contains large amounts of unhealthy saturated fat. Margarine is not a healthy alternative – it often contains trans-fat and artificial ingredients.

Omega-3 fatty acids are a family of essential polyunsaturated fats.

- ◊ These essential fatty acids are not made by the body and must be obtained in food.
- ◊ They include eicosapentaenoic acid (EPA) and docosahexaenoic acid (DHA), both derivates of alpha-linoleic acid (ALA). They are found in the oils of cold water fish.
- ◊ EPA plays a role in cardiovascular health, while DHA is important for the neurologic system.[14]
- ◊ They have **anti-inflammatory and anti-thrombotic** properties. They are incorporated into cell membranes and decrease synthesis of prostaglandins, thromboxane A2, and leukotrienes.
- ◊ Ancestral diets contained high amounts of the omega-3 fatty acids due to high intake of whole plant foods and absence of processed foods and meats. Today's western diet contains more pro-inflammatory (omega-6) fatty acids.
- ◊ To obtain omega-3 fatty acids, fish consumption is preferred over fish oil supplements. However, if supplementing fish oil, consume 1000-2000 mg/day and look for quantities of 200-500mg DHA and 700-1000mg EPA.
- ◊ Vegetarian sources include walnuts, flaxseed, chia seeds, hemp seed and milk.

Does a low-fat diet promote weight loss?

- ◊ This diet fails to recognize the importance of healthy fats. For example, the Mediterranean diet contains high amounts of healthy fat and is associated with *lower* risk of obesity.
- ◊ Patients on a low-fat diet often rely on processed "non-fat" or "low-fat" snack foods, frozen dinners, and yogurts that are empty of nutrients and contain added sugars. For example, *Reduced Fat* Oreos contain less fat (4.5 g) but still contain 13g of sugar per serving as well as artificial ingredients.
- ◊ Instead, focus on increasing vegetable and fruit intake and limiting processed food and meat.

Sample Healthy Portion Sizes (up to once a day)

◊ Avocado: quarter-size chunk
◊ Walnuts: two nuts
◊ Almonds: ¼ cup, or 7-10 nuts
◊ Olive oil: ½ tablespoon (salad dressing for one person, 1-2 tablespoons (sautéing)
◊ Whole fat Greek yogurt: ¼ to ½ cup

Fats – Bottom Line

◊ Reduce saturated and trans-fat by avoiding processed meat, processed snack foods, and fast food.
◊ Include healthy fats – olive and plant oils, nuts, and avocados (just watch portions).
◊ Substitute olive oil for butter in cooking. Avoid margarine and shortening.
◊ Try plain Greek yogurt for shortening, cream, and butter on baked potatoes and in baked goods.
◊ Consume fish (organic, wild and not farmed, when possible) if you eat meat.

CARBOHYDRATES – *QUALITY MATTERS*

- ◊ Carbohydrates can be divided into refined carbohydrates and complex carbohydrates.
- ◊ Refined carbs are in processed foods – white or enriched breads and pastas, white rice, sugary cereals, baked goods, cookies, and crackers.
- ◊ Complex carbs are in whole foods – whole grains, peas, beans, and vegetables.
- ◊ **Complex carbs have more fiber and plant-based protein, promoting satiety.** They also have a lower glycemic impact (see below).
- ◊ Glycemic Index and Glycemic Load – *the lower, the better*.
    - o Glycemic index (GI) – a measure of how high the blood sugar rises after consuming a given serving of a food.
    - o Glycemic load (GL) – similar to GI, but also accounts for the amount of carbohydrate in the food. More predictive of the glycemic impact of food than GI.
    - o GI and GL can differ significantly. For example – carrots (GI of 35, GL of 2).

Glycemic impact of sample foods[15]

Food	GI	GL
White bread, slice	73	10
Whole wheat bread, slice	71	9
Whole grain bread, slice	51	7
White bagel	72	25
White rice	89	43
Brown rice	50	16
Carrots, 1 cup	35	2
Apple juice	44	30
Banana	62	16
Fruit Roll-up	99	24
Clif Bar	101	49

- Incorporating certain foods into a meal can lower glycemic load.
    - **Vinegar** (consumed before a meal) – due to acetic acid content.[16]
    - **Cinnamon** – contains a compound that mimics insulin.[17]
    - **Fiber** also lowers the glycemic load of a meal.
- Low GI/GL foods help prevent insulin resistance and are associated with better glycemic control in diabetics.

Does a low-carb diet promote weight loss?
- This diet fails to recognize that complex carbs can actually aid weight loss!
- Instead, focus on avoiding processed foods and refined carbs.

Carbohydrates – Bottom line

- Avoid processed foods and sugar-sweetened beverages.
- Consider whole grains (quinoa, barley, etc.) as the main protein source for a meal.
- Tropical fruits and bananas have the highest glycemic load of all fruits. Choose more berries, nectarines, apples, pears, and oranges/grapefruits.
- Consider a salad with balsamic vinegar or apple cider vinegar before a meal.
- Sprinkle cinnamon into soups, flat breads, and oatmeal to lower glycemic load. It may add a touch of sweetness or be unnoticed.

WHOLE GRAINS

◊ The fiber in whole grains absorbs water and expands. As a general rule, you know they are done when the overlying water disappears, and they are moist and fluffy.
◊ Most can be cooked in an uncovered saucepan. Rice and quinoa are fluffier when cooked with the lid on.

Whole grain	Grain	Water	Instructions	Uses
Rolled oats	1 cup	2 cups	Combine and bring to a boil; simmer 10-15 min.	Breakfast oatmeal; baking (cookies, muffins); granola bars
Steel cut oats	1 cup	4 cups	Combine and bring to a boil; simmer 30 min.	Breakfast oatmeal
Brown rice	1 cup	2 cups	Combine and bring to a boil; simmer covered 35-45 min.; avoid stirring.	Substitute for white rice in stir-fries (short grain) and pilaf (long grain)
Quinoa	1 cup	2 cups	Rinse quinoa in sieve. Combine with water and boil; simmer covered 20 min; fluff with fork.	Lunch/dinner with veggies; veggie burgers; breakfast porridge
Bulgur	1 cup	2 ½ cups	Combine and bring to a boil; simmer 20-25 min.	Substitute for quinoa; tabouli and other salads
Buckwheat	1 cup	~3 cups	Add buckwheat to pot and cover with water; boil until oats are soft. Drain excess water.	Breakfast porridge; toasted in granola
Barley	1 cup	3 ½ cups	Combine and bring to a boil; simmer 50-60 min.	Breakfast porridge; substitute for rice in risotto and rice salads
Popcorn			Heat 2-3 tbsp oil on medium-high heat. Add single layer of kernels; cover; shake pot continuously.	A great snack
Millet	1 cup	2 ½ cups	Combine and bring to a boil; simmer 20-25 min.	Substitute for quinoa; breakfast porridge; millet bread

PROTEIN – *THE PLANT-BASED WAY*

The optimal protein intake for adults may vary based on age, sex, and activity level; however, the general recommendations are 0.8g/kg daily (56g for a 70kg man) or 10-35% of calories.[18,19] Many Americans eat an excessive amount of protein, especially in low quality and processed meats.

In fact, protein can be found in a variety of plant foods –

- ◊ **Nuts**
    - o Peanuts – ¼ cup = 8g
    - o Almonds – ¼ cup = 6g
    - o Pumpkin seeds – ¼ cup = 7g
- ◊ **Grains**
    - o Brown rice – 1 cup cooked = 6g
    - o Quinoa – 1 cup cooked = 9g
- ◊ **Legumes**
    - o Beans (black beans, kidney beans) – 1 cup = 15g
    - o Lentils – 1 cup = 18g
    - o Garbanzos/chickpeas – 1 cup = 12g
- ◊ **Green peas** – 1 cup = 8g
- ◊ **Soy** (edamame, tofu, tempeh) – 1 serving = 20g
- ◊ **Chia seeds** – 2 tablespoons = 6g

Other non-meat sources of protein –
- ◊ **Eggs** (organic when possible) – 1 egg = 6g
- ◊ **Greek yogurt** (organic; be aware of sugar content) – 1 cup = 17g
- ◊ **Tuna, salmon** – ½ can = 20g

What about iron?

- There are two types of iron – heme iron (found in meat and fish) and nonheme iron (found in plants).
- Because nonheme iron is less bioavailable, vegetarians are more susceptible to low iron stores.[20,21] Vegetarians should double their iron intake from plant-based sources. These include whole grains, beans, lentils, tofu, cocoa powder, and dark chocolate.
- There is evidence that heme iron, found especially in red meat, contributes to the development of type 2 diabetes and heart disease.[22] Vegetarians have lower rates of both conditions.

Protein – Bottom line

- Protein is satiating and can help with weight maintenance if consumed from healthy sources.
- Unless you are an elite athlete or engage in strenuous exercise daily, you probably don't need extra protein.
- Protein can be found in a variety of plant foods.
- Limit red and processed meat.

COOKING AT HOME

In a culture of processed and fast food, most Americans are no longer connected to where our food comes from and how it is made. Cooking encourages us to think about what goes into our bodies. It is an opportunity to have fun, be creative, relieve stress and save money. It can be a family activity or a meditative solo practice. When we create our own nutritious meals from scratch, fast food and processed food become less desirable. In fact, a recent study shows that food is perceived to taste better when we prepare it ourselves.[23]

Did you know?

- Cooking pasta *al dente* (cooked for less time so it is firm to the bite) lowers its glycemic impact.
- Heating garlic alters much of its health benefits, including anti-cancer properties. Preserve its health benefits by chopping it and letting it sit for 10 to 15 minutes before heating.[24]

Cooking tips

- Stock your kitchen! (See "Plant-based kitchen staples" below.)
- Cook using basic ingredients ("from scratch") as much as possible.
- Avoid frying, overcooking or charring meat. Avoid processed meats (bacon, sausage, salami, hot dogs).
- Use olive oil or coconut oil instead of butter.
- Avoid butter/margarine and cream-based sauces and cheese, especially on vegetables.
- Replace salt in recipes with herbs and spices. If needed, add salt to taste with a salt shaker.
- Cook with whole grains such as brown rice and quinoa, and use whole-wheat pasta.

How to: Roast vegetables

What to roast: Root vegetables (potatoes, sweet potatoes, carrots), broccoli and cauliflower, zucchini, bell peppers, tomatoes, onions, garlic, brussel sprouts, beets
*Note: Roast veggies with similar cooking times together (root vegetables take longer).

How: Chop veggies and place in large bowl. Toss with olive oil (enough to coat but not soak). Add a teaspoon of salt and black pepper, and herbs if desired (thyme, rosemary, oregano). Toss and spread evenly in one layer on a baking sheet. Bake at 425 degrees F for about 30 minutes, until you see some char on the edges, checking every 15 minutes.

Use in pasta, salads, pizzas, sandwiches, and quinoa.

PLANT-BASED KITCHEN STAPLES

These are versatile and can be used in many easy recipes.

- ◊ **Vegetables** - the more colorful, the better
    - o Cruciferous vegetables – broccoli, brussels sprouts, cauliflower – have anticancer properties
    - o Leafy greens – kale, spinach, collard greens
    - o Flavorful micro greens – cilantro, parsley, basil
    - o Other colorful vegetables – peppers and eggplant

- ◊ **Fruits**
    - o Berries – full of antioxidants; buy frozen to save money
    - o Apples - buy organic if possible
    - o Bananas - inexpensive, although higher glycemic index

- ◊ **Plant-based protein**
    - o Soy – fermented (miso and tempeh), soybeans, tofu
    - o Plain Greek yogurt (plain)
    - o Lentils, beans, and chickpeas – dried or canned
    - o Eggs – cage-free, organic if possible

- ◊ **Plant-based milk** – buy unsweetened to avoid excess sugar
    - o Almond milk, hemp milk, soy milk, rice milk

- ◊ **Grains**
    - o Oats – steel-cut are the most healthful, followed by rolled oats and then instant/quick oats
    - o Brown rice, quinoa, bulgur, barley

- **Frozen**
    - Berries
    - Peas, edamame
    - Vegetables – frozen vegetables only lose 10% of their nutrients!

- **Spices/oils**
    - Olive oil – extra-virgin, expeller-pressed, organic, local if possible; and/or coconut oil
    - Vinegar – lowers glycemic impact of meals
    - Soy sauce/tamari (low sodium), sesame oil
    - Anti-inflammatory herbs/spices – ginger, cumin, cayenne, turmeric, dried basil, oregano, thyme

- **Occasionally** – watch portions
    - Wild salmon
    - Lean meat – organic if possible – skinless chicken breast, turkey, bison

> **Did you know?**
> Different oils have different smoke points, that is, the temperature at which they smoke and release harmful free radicals. A higher smoke point is ideal for an oil you heat and cook with. For example, olive oil has a moderately high smoke point and is good for sautéing. Extra virgin olive oil has a slightly lower smoke point and is good for salad dressings. Learn more about smoke points of oils at mayoclinig.org.

> Frozen berries are cheaper, last longer, and have **just as many antioxidants** as fresh berries.[25]

FOOD COMPARISONS

It is possible to replace processed foods with whole foods without compromising taste. Other simple ingredient swaps can help eliminate harmful ingredients from your diet – for example, substitute Greek yogurt for mayonnaise. Make your own breadcrumbs by toasting whole grain bread and processing in a food processor!

- ◊ **Butter/spreads**[26]
    - Least healthy – margarine – *often high amounts of trans fat*
    - Not healthy – butter – *high amounts of saturated fat*
    - Somewhat healthy – new vegetable-based spreads such as Earth Balance – *mostly unsaturated fat, but still high calorie*
    - Healthiest – olive oil, Greek yogurt, unsweetened applesauce (in baked goods)
- ◊ **Flour**
    - Least healthy – white flour – *in the process of milling into white flour, whole wheat flour loses several plant-based nutrients*
    - Somewhat healthy – whole wheat flour - *although roughly the same glycemic index as white flour*
    - Healthiest – chickpea flour, almond flour, brown rice flour

> ### Recipe: Dijon vinaigrette
>
> Combine 1 tbsp Dijon mustard, ¼ cup red wine vinegar or apple cider vinegar, ¼ cup extra virgin olive oil, 1 teaspoon honey, 1 tablespoon fresh lemon juice, and salt and pepper or herbs to taste.

- ◊ **Salad dressing**
    - Least healthy – store-bought Ranch, bleu cheese, and other creamy dressings
    - Not healthy – store bought "no-fat", or "low-fat" dressings – *often contain artificial ingredients and hidden sugar*
    - Somewhat healthy – store-bought vinaigrette
    - Healthiest (and cheapest!) – homemade vinaigrette

- ◊ **Fruit**
    - Least healthy – canned/packaged fruit in syrup
    - Healthier – canned fruit in its own juices
    - Healthiest – fresh, whole fruit
    - Just as healthy – frozen fruit

> A 6oz portion of **plain** Greek yogurt contains 4-7 grams of sugar naturally. One small container of 0% **blueberry** yogurt contains **15g** of sugar. That's 8g of added sugar (2 teaspoons)!

- ◊ **Yogurt**
    - Least healthy – flavored yogurt with added sugars
    - Not healthy – "fat-free" flavored yogurt – *usually contains artificial ingredients and added sugars*
    - Healthiest – plain Greek yogurt – *add fresh fruit, cinnamon, or a touch of honey for sweetness*
    - Tips
        - Eat a smaller portion size if eating whole fat yogurt.
        - Look for less than 9 grams of sugar per serving (6oz or 1 cup).

- **Lettuce**
    - Least healthy – iceberg lettuce – *low in nutrients*
    - Healthier – romaine, spring mix/mesclun
    - Healthiest – dark, leafy greens – kale, collards, spinach, arugula, Asian greens

- **Fruit drinks/smoothies**
    - Least healthy – most prepared smoothies at restaurants and "smoothie bars" – *large amounts of sugar; often ice cream/sorbet*
    - Somewhat healthy – bottled fruit drinks (Odwalla, Naked Juice) – *large amounts of sugar; usually no protein or fiber*
    - Healthy – homemade smoothie with greens and fresh or frozen fruit, with optional plain Greek yogurt
    - Healthiest – whole green leafy vegetables and fruits

- **Cereal**
    - While unprocessed oats and other whole grains are ideal, cereal can be a healthy breakfast option.[27]
    - Look for **less than 6 grams** of sugar. Add fresh or dried fruit for sweetness.
    - Look for at least 3-4 grams of protein and at least 3 grams of fiber.
    - Check the box for whole grains (**at least 16 grams** per serving). The first ingredients listed should be whole grain oats or whole wheat.
    - Be mindful of store-bought granola, which may be high in fat and sugar content. Note that the serving size is small (about ½ cup).
    - Try unsweetened, plant-based milk such as almond milk.

CEREAL COMPARISONS

Cereal	Sugar (grams)	Fiber (g)	Protein (g)	Whole grains (g)
Cheerios (General Mill's)	1	3	3	14
Trader Joe's Multigrain O's	6	3	2	14
Shredded Wheat (Arrowhead Mills)	2	6	6	40
Heritage Bites (Nature's Path)	3	5	3	18
Wheat Squares (Whole Foods 365)	0	5	4	49
Wheaties (General Mills)	4	3	2	22
Uncle Sam Original	<1	10	7	43
Go Lean Crunch! (Kashi)	13	8	9	19
Corn Flakes (Kellogg's)	3	1	2	0
Frosted Flakes (Kellogg's)	11	<1	1	0
Special K (Kellogg's)	4	0	6	0
Raisin Bran (Kellogg's)	18	7	4	27

Look for the whole grains label when buying cereal, and aim for at least 16g per serving.
Image: wholegrainscouncil.org

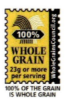 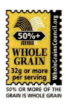 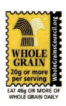

PRACTICAL HEALTHY MEAL SWAPS

Make veggies and grains the main part of your meal, with fish or other meat as an optional side dish.

Breakfast
- ◊ Less healthy option: Cheese omelet with bacon/sausage; white toast or home-fries
    - o Healthier alternative: Veggie omelet with broccoli, spinach, tomato, mushrooms, and optional cheese. Add a side of roasted sweet potatoes, steel-cut oats or whole grain toast.
- ◊ Less healthy option: Plain bagel with cream cheese
    - o Healthier alternative: Whole grain toast with peanut butter and banana. *Sprinkle cinnamon to lower glycemic impact.*
- ◊ Less healthy option: Waffles with syrup
    - o Healthier alternative: Whole-grain, chickpea flour, or sweet potato pancakes with fresh fruit

Lunch
- ◊ Less healthy option: Fried chicken sandwich on white bun; french fries
    - o Healthier alternative: Whole grain bread with avocado, smashed chickpeas, tomato, and raw spinach; optional chicken breast
    - o For another healthy alternative see *Quinoa with veggies* in the Recipes section!
- ◊ Less healthy option: Slice of pepperoni pizza
    - o Healthier alternative: Large salad with carrots, tomatoes, nuts, and olive oil vinaigrette. Add a slice of vegetable pizza. *Sprinkle flaxseed for omega-3 antioxidants and fiber.*

Dinner
- ◊ Less healthy option: Baked ziti or meat lasagna (white pasta noodles, ground meat, cheese, and pasta sauce)
    - o Healthier alternative: Pasta primavera – whole-wheat spaghetti, cooked al dente, with vegetables (broccoli, asparagus, mushroom, tomato, spinach). Add fresh garlic oregano, or thyme to increase anti-inflammatory benefit.

HEALTHY ON A BUDGET

Eating healthy doesn't have to be expensive, especially when you cook at home. Even organic, plant-based nutrition can be affordable with careful meal planning.
To save time and money, cook in batches for the week and pack leftovers for lunch. For the best deals on produce, stop by the farmer's market for local produce that is in season.

Even superfoods have cheaper alternatives –

- **Quinoa – full of protein and fiber** – 8 g protein, 5 g fiber per cup ($5-8 per pound)
    - Brown rice – 5 g protein, 3.5 g fiber ($1-2 per pound)
    - Lentils – 18 g protein, 16 g fiber ($1-2 per pound)
    - Millet – 6 g protein, 2 g fiber ($2 per pound)
    - Bulgur wheat – 6 g protein, 8 g fiber ($2-4 per pound)

- **Walnuts – rich in anti-inflammatory omega-3's** ($7-13 per pound)
    - Roasted chickpeas – 15 g protein and 12 g fiber per cup ($1 per can!)
    - Peanuts – 7 g protein per serving; rich in Vitamin E ($3 per pound)
    - Almonds – 4 g fiber per serving ($6-11 per pound)

> **Consider this –**
> - The most expensive food is the food we waste! The US alone wastes **billions of dollars** in discarded food annually.
> - Americans spend **billions** of dollars on bottled water annually, while many countries lack access to drinkable water.[28]

ORGANIC FOOD: AN INVESTMENT TOWARD YOUR HEALTH

◊ Organic produce contains approximately four times less pesticide residue than conventional crops, and 20-70% greater concentrations of disease-fighting antioxidants.[29]

◊ Despite the health risks inherent to pesticide use, there have been few studies demonstrating the health benefit of organic food.[30]

◊ In general, organic crops are considered safer for the environment and harvesters. Pesticide exposure may even contribute to cancer risk in humans.[31]

◊ **Organic does not always mean healthy!** While fresh organic produce may be healthier, processed foods made with "organic" ingredients may still contain high amounts of sugar, unhealthy fat, and salt.

◊ Eating organic can be more costly, making it less feasible for some budgets. Some foods may be more worth the cost than others[32]– the environmental working group comes out with recommendations on an annual basis, per www.ewg.org.

Dirty dozen – may contain more pesticides and should be bought organic.
- Fruit – strawberries, apples, nectarines and peaches, grapes, cherries,
- Vegetables – celery, tomatoes/cherry tomatoes, bell peppers, cucumbers, spinach

Clean fifteen – Often contain skins that are removed; can be bought non-organic.
- Fruit - avocado, pineapple, mango, papaya, kiwi, grapefruit, honeydew, cantaloupe
- Vegetables - cabbage, frozen sweet peas, cauliflower, onions, corn

> ### Washing produce
>
> ◊ All produce should be washed, including organic produce.
> ◊ **Water** (lukewarm or cold) is an effective rinse for fruits/vegetables.
> ◊ Fruit and vegetable washes have not been investigated thoroughly and are not recommended by the FDA. Studies show they are no more effective at killing bacteria than water.[33]
> ◊ Other tips[34]
>   o Wait to wash produce until you are going to consume it (avoid pre-washing).
>   o There is no need to re-wash pre-washed lettuce or other vegetables.
>   o Use a produce brush for produce with thick/bumpy skin or rinds, such as potatoes.
>   o To wash mushrooms, rub them with a wet paper towel or clean washcloth.

Compare the additional cost of organic food to some unnecessary expenses[35] –

◊ Green bell peppers (1 pound) - conventional $1.50, organic $2.75
  o Cost difference of $1.25 = 1 gallon of bottled water
◊ Strawberries (1 pound) - conventional $3.99, organic $4.50
  o Cost difference of $1.50 = 1 can of soda in vending machine
◊ Milk (one gallon) - conventional $4, organic $6.50
  o Cost difference of $2.50 = large bag of snack mix
◊ Eggs (one dozen) - conventional $3, organic $4.75
  o Cost difference of $1.75 = pack of gum
◊ Black beans (1 can) - conventional $0.99, organic $1.40
◊ Apples (1 pound) - conventional $1.50, organic $2.50
◊ Frozen chicken breasts (1 pound) - conventional $3.50, organic $5.00
◊ Lettuce (1 head) - conventional $2, organic $4

> Extra cost of buying 1 pound of organic strawberries per week versus conventional, for 1 year = $25

Be wary of food labels! With the increased popularity of organic foods, some large companies market food as organic without meeting standards.[36]

◊ **Trust these labels** –
- 100% organic
- Organic (USDA Organic)
- "Made with organic ingredients" – at least 70% of ingredients are organic

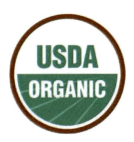

- **Don't trust these labels –**

    - "Free-range", "free-roaming" (eggs and chicken) – means that animals are allowed out of cages for a *portion* of the day, which could be only 5 minutes!

    - "Natural" or "all-natural" – claim is not standardized nor verified.

    - "Natural flavoring" – used to describe any product used for flavoring that is *derived* from a natural product.[37] Does not mean that the product does not contain artificial ingredients.

> While plant-based milk is a better option for our health and for animal well-being, for those who drink dairy milk, organic may be a healthier option than conventional. It contains more omega-3 fatty acids[38], likely because organic cows usually feed on their natural diet of grass rather than genetically modified corn and soy feed.
>
> Organic meat also has more omega-3s than conventional meat.

PART TWO: HEALTHY EATING

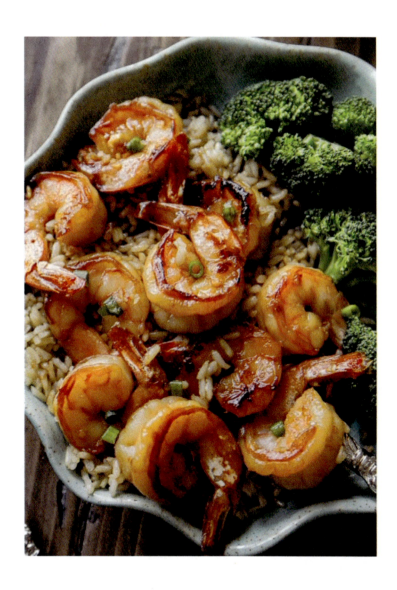

THE ANTI-INFLAMMATORY APPROACH TO EATING

Chronic inflammation may lead to disease by impairing the body's own healing processes. Factors contributing to inflammation include stress and lack of exercise. Nutrition also plays a vital role, as certain foods (such as mushrooms and berries) fight inflammation. The anti-inflammatory diet, made popular by integrative medicine pioneer Dr. Andrew Weil, emphasizes[39] –

- ◊ Vegetables – at least 4 servings per day, especially cruciferous
- ◊ Fruits – at least 3 servings per day, especially non-tropical fruits
- ◊ Fiber – goal of 40 grams per day
- ◊ Whole grains
- ◊ Pasta cooked *al dente*
- ◊ Healthy fats – extra virgin olive oil, omega-3 fats from fish and soy
- ◊ Plant-based protein – whole grains, soy, beans
- ◊ Other protein – 1-2 servings per week of lean skinless chicken, organic eggs, natural cheese
- ◊ Fish – wild salmon and herring
- ◊ Mushrooms – cooked Asian mushrooms, such as shitake, maitake, oyster, cordiceps
- ◊ Anti-inflammatory herbs and spices – turmeric, curry, rosemary, ginger, garlic, chili, basil
- ◊ Sweets – sparingly – dark chocolate and unsweetened dried fruit
- ◊ Tea – high quality green, white, oolong teas – *have the most antioxidants*
- ◊ Red wine – occasionally – *red grapes contain the same antioxidant (resveratrol)*

Anti-inflammatory spices

A recent study showed that certain spices have an anti-inflammatory effect. A significantly reduced inflammatory response was noted in the blood plasma of participants who consumed **cloves, ginger, rosemary,** or **turmeric**.[40]

The anti-inflammatory food pyramid:

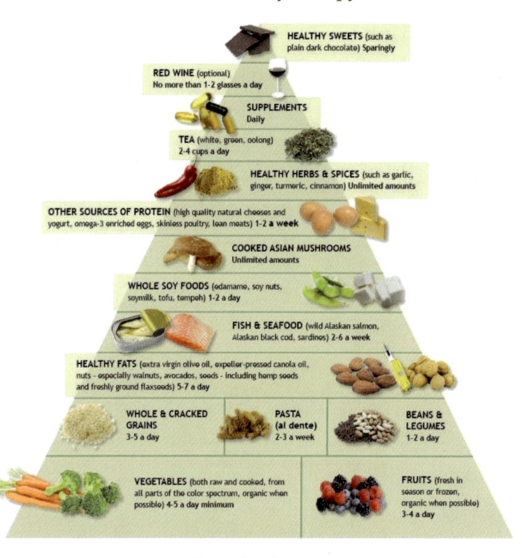

Image: drweil.com

VITAMINS: SHOULD I TAKE THEM?

Vitamins are essential for normal growth and maintenance. They are required in *small* quantities in the diet. Fat soluble vitamins (A, D, E, K) are stored in the body more readily than water-soluble vitamins. Roughly half of the US population reports taking a dietary supplement such as a daily multivitamin. However, vitamin supplementation is intended for special patient populations, and overall Americans take too many vitamins and supplements.

- Several studies have found no benefit to the average person from the use of vitamins, and some have shown potential harm.[41] For example, excess B6 can cause neuropathy, and excess Vitamin A and E have been associated with cancer, headache, and spinal cord issues.
- **The US Preventative Services Task Force (USPSTF) has concluded that there is insufficient evidence for using multivitamins or nutrient supplements to prevent cardiovascular disease and cancer.**
- Dietary supplements, including vitamins, are not FDA regulated. Therefore it is not required that they are proven safe and effective before entering the market.
- If buying vitamins, check for the USP label "high quality" for quality assurance.

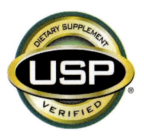

Image: wholefoodsmarket.com

VITAMIN D

Despite evidence for the importance of Vitamin D, supplementation remains a contested topic.

◊ Vitamin D is made by the skin when it is exposed to sunlight.

◊ Vitamin D deficiency has been linked to health problems including multiple sclerosis, cancer, autoimmune disease, chronic pain syndrome, cardiac disease, and diabetes.

◊ Many Americans are Vitamin D deficient due to more time spent indoors and use of sunblock, which blocks up to 99% of conversion to active form.

◊ A study in the Journal of Pediatrics found that 70% of US children and adolescents ages 1-21 were not getting enough Vitamin D.[42]

◊ Most experts agree that 25-hydroxy-vitamin D serum concentrations of 30-40 ng/mL are sufficient. Concentrations <20 mg/dL may negatively impact bone health.

◊ **A recent meta-analysis concluded that the evidence is severely lacking for vitamin D supplementation in the general, healthy population.**[43]

PATIENT GUIDANCE

TRANSITIONING FROM SELF-CARE TO PATIENT COUNSELING

The doctor of the future will give no medicine, but will interest her or his patients in the care of the human frame, **in a proper diet***, and in the cause and prevention of disease.*

-Thomas Edison (1847-1931)

Counseling patients on healthy eating requires more than just nutrition knowledge. Many patients face barriers to healthy eating, such as lack of access to affordable produce or cultural influences on food and body. Others may lack the confidence or motivation to change their eating habits. Society, family and friend circles, and work life are powerful influences on food choices. Media is also important – we are not only daily consumers of food, but also of advertising. The media promotes sugary, salty food, as well as quick and easy weight loss solutions – it is not uncommon for patients to have tried several "fad" diets.

Physicians play a powerful role in guiding patients to make better choices. **When contemplating the time it takes to discuss nutrition with a patient, compare it to the time spent providing counseling on medication regimens and monitoring for adverse reactions.** Changing the food we eat is a long-lasting treatment that is easy to prescribe with minimal cost and side effects.

MOTIVATIONAL INTERVIEWING

◊ Motivational interviewing is a patient-centered counseling style used to promote behavior change in patients who feel ambivalent. It has been used successfully in addiction counseling.

- Key principles of motivational interviewing[44] –
    - Emphasizes patient self-direction, with provider guidance as needed.
    - Identifies barriers to change.
    - Uses a collaborative approach.
    - Emphasizes empathy from provider rather than confrontation.
    - Supports patient's self-efficacy and confidence in change.

◊ Based on a 2011 meta-analysis, motivational interviewing appears to be an effective tool to encourage weight loss in obese patients.[45]

◊ Useful tools[46]
- **Elicit desire** for behavior change
    - "Is there anything you would like to do for your health in the next week/month?"
    Physician can make suggestions if patient needs help ("If it's helpful I can share some ideas...")
- **Collaborate on a plan**
    - Clarify what, where, when, and how often
    - Commitment statement - "To make sure we both understand, could you tell me again what you've decided to do?"

- **Assess confidence**

    - "I would like to know how confident you feel about carrying out your plan. On a scale of 0 to 10, where 0 means you are not at all confident and 10 means you are very confident, about how confident do you feel?" *Physician may use hands as an imaginary ruler.*
    - If confidence is <7, talk about overcoming barriers or adjusting the plan. Physician might say, "A 5 is great - much higher than 0! I wonder if there is any way we might adjust the plan to get you to a 7 or higher. Maybe we could make the goal a little easier, or you could ask for help from friends."

- **Change talk** – Prompt the patient to describe his motivations and readiness for change. Help the patient to realize the discrepancy between his values and behavior. Elicit change talk with these questions –

    - What might you enjoy about eating healthier?
    - If you decided to eat healthier, how would you do it?
    - How important is it to you to eat healthier?
    - What are the most important reasons you see for eating healthier?
    - What are you already doing to make it possible to eat healthier?

- **Arrange follow-up** – create accountability
    - "That sounds like a plan that's going to work for you. When would you like to check in with me to review how you're doing with your plan?"

SAMPLE DIALOGUE

Below is an example of how a motivational interviewing session might proceed. *Written by Jessica Deffler.*

- Doctor (D): Is there anything you would like to do for your health in the next month?
- Patient (P): I'm not quite sure, doctor. I already have a lot on my plate with my diabetes and high blood pressure.
- D: I understand. It must be difficult to keep up with all of the medications and doctor visits. If you don't have any ideas, perhaps we can talk about nutrition. Would you mind if I ask you some questions about what you like to eat?
- P: Sure, that is fine.
- D: Great. Tell me what sorts of things you like to eat.
- P: Well, I usually don't eat breakfast because I wake up so early. If I'm lucky to get a break at work I grab lunch at one of the fast food places nearby. After work I eat whatever my wife makes for dinner at home.
- D: I see. Is there anything you are doing to try to change how you eat, or eat healthier?
- P: Not especially. My heart doctor tells me I should try to cut out fats.
- D: Can you think of any reasons why you would like to eat healthier? (What might you enjoy about eating healthier? How important is it to you to eat healthier?)
- P: Well, I think it would help me lose some of this weight. I've been having trouble keeping up with my sons lately...I get short of breath and I think maybe it's this weight I've put on.
- D: It must be difficult not being able to keep up with your sons – I think that's a great reason to make some changes. Just eating healthier will help you feel better, too, regardless of your weight.
- P: I think so, too.
- D: If you decided to eat healthier, how do you think you would do it?
- P: Well, like I said, I usually eat what my wife cooks for dinner, so I can't really change that. I guess I could change what I eat for lunch, though.
- D: I think that's a good start. Tell me more about how you could do that.

- P: Well, I usually go to a fast food place because I don't get much time on my break. Maybe I could try to find a healthier place like a smoothie shop or something.
- D: It sounds like you are willing to limit fast food, which is great. I think another great option is packing a lunch. How do you feel about that?
- P: I guess I could do that, but I'm not sure I would have time.
- D: I understand. Maybe we can talk about tips for cooking ahead of time so that you can pack a lunch easily. Or if you'd prefer, we can talk more about other healthier options for eating out.
- P: I think I'd be willing to try packing a lunch.
- D: I'm glad to hear that. Packing your lunch will allow you to know exactly what you're eating, control your portion sizes, and save money, too. *<Provides specific foods and tips for packing a lunch.>*
- P: That sounds good. I think I could do that.
- D: Would you like to set a goal for yourself for before the next time I see you?
- P: Well, I think I could start packing my lunch every day.
- D: I think that sounds good. We all know that changing a behavior is very difficult, so I'm wondering if you could tell me how confident you feel that you will be able to achieve your goal. On a scale of 1 to 10, how confident are you? *<Holds up an imaginary ruler with hands.>*
- P: (Patient points) I think probably around here, a 5.
- D: A 5 is a start, much higher than a 0! I wonder if we can get you even more confident with achieving your goal, if we make the goal more achievable - for example, you can try to pack your lunch twice a week at first.
- P: I think I could do three times a week, definitely. My confidence is about a 7 or 8 then.
- D: That sounds better to me. We can slowly work up to every day. I'm confident that you will be able to achieve your goal, and I'm here to support you.
- P: Thanks, doctor.
- D: When would you like me to check in with you to see how you are doing with your goal?
- P: I think after two weeks would be good, I can call the office to update you.

BARRIERS TO HEALTHY EATING

◊ Lack of healthy food access (especially in food deserts*)
◊ Cultural influences on food and body type
◊ Work environment
◊ Family dynamics/preferences
◊ Preconceptions on the cost of healthy food
◊ Lack of basic nutrition knowledge

*A **food desert** is an area of the country with very little access to fresh produce and other whole foods. Usually found in impoverished areas lacking grocery stores and farmers markets.

The USDA defines a food desert as an area in which at least one-third of residents live more than 1 mile away from fresh food (or 10 miles in a rural area).[47]

PART THREE: DIET AND DISEASE

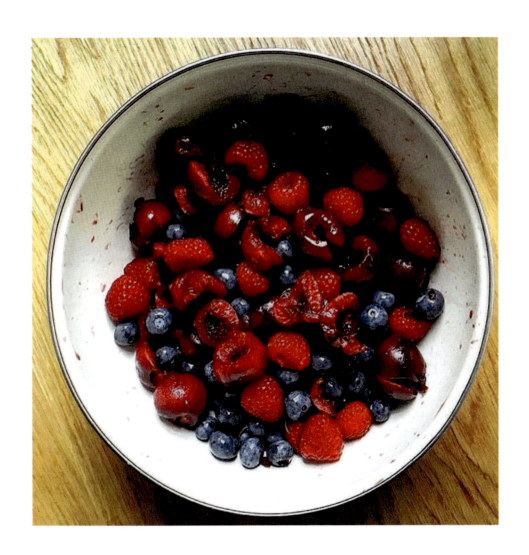

DIET & DISEASE: EVIDENCE-BASED NUTRITION AS MEDICINE

"Most deaths in the United States are preventable, and they are related to what we eat."
– Michael Greger, MD, *How Not to Die*

Plant-based, whole food nutrition can prevent disease.

Obesity
- Practice intuitive eating.
- Replace simple sugars and refined carbs with complex carbs.
- Eat mostly "energy dilute foods" – foods that satiate with high water and fiber content.

Heart disease
- Limit red meat and processed meat to limit unhealthy saturated fat and other harmful ingredients.
- Reduce use of creamy sauces, dressings, and butter.
- Consume healthy nuts in small portions.

Diabetes
- ◊ Even modest weight loss (10%) is beneficial.
- ◊ Fiber and healthy unsaturated fats improve glycemic control.
- ◊ Decrease use of all sweeteners.

Cancer
- ◊ Limit red and processed meats. Choose lean meats preferably.
- ◊ Consume antioxidant-rich fruits and vegetables.

Hypertension
- ◊ Limit meat, especially red and processed meat.
- ◊ Use salt sparingly, reading food labels for sodium content.
- ◊ Avoid excess alcohol.

Gastrointestinal Disease
- ◊ Patients with Celiac disease should avoid gluten.
- ◊ Irritable Bowel Syndrome or non-celiac gluten sensitivity may improve with a gluten-free or low-FODMAP diet, and increased fiber intake.
- ◊ Consume both probiotics and prebiotics.

Neurologic Disease
- ◊ Headaches may be triggered by certain foods.
- ◊ A food diary helps to identify triggers.
- ◊ Antioxidant intake in fruits and vegetables over time may help maintain brain and nerve health while preventing cognitive decline with aging.

OBESITY

"Competing diet claims are diverting attention and resources from what is actually and urgently needed: a dedicated and concerted effort to make the basic dietary pattern known to support both health and weight control more accessible to all." –
David Katz, MD, *Nutrition in Clinical Practice*

While genetics explain 40% of weight variation, environment is the main contributor to the obesity epidemic. Obesity is a major risk factor for Type 2 diabetes, heart disease, and cancer. In particular, central or abdominal obesity is associated with metabolic syndrome, diabetes, cardiovascular disease, and mortality.

Healthy nutrition prevents obesity and its associated chronic diseases. There are several barriers to preventing obesity, including poverty, food access, and marketing. Despite these obstacles, we can make an impact by educating ourselves and counseling our patients.

> Waist circumference and waist-to-hip ratio predict mortality better than Body Mass Index.[48]

WEIGHT LOSS – BASIC APPROACH

◊ The simple math of "calories in, calories out" holds true for weight loss. To lose weight, one either has to consume less calories or burn more. *Caloric requirements for weight maintenance/loss can be calculated with the Harris-Benedict equation (available at users.med.cornell.edu).*

◊ Yet, **not all calories are created equal.** Different foods produce a different amount of fullness for a given number of calories, depending on their water, fiber, and protein content.

- o *Energy dilute* foods provide satiety with fewer calories. They include vegetables and fruits with high water and fiber content.
- o *Energy dense* foods contain more calories per bite and lead to greater calorie consumption to provide satiety. They include fast food and snack foods with high fat and sugar content.
- o Consuming an array of energy dilute foods promotes weight loss without overly restricting ones diet.

◊ Basal metabolic rate (BMR) = resting metabolic rate + energy burned

- o An individual's BMR is largely explained by lean body mass, although it varies based on age and sex.
- o Depending on BMR, a given caloric intake can produce weight gain in some individuals but not others (i.e., some individuals are "predisposed" to weight gain.)
- o Weight loss reduces BMR, so that maintenance of weight loss becomes more difficult after early success.[1]
- o Exercise can help build lean body mass, maintaining ones BMR while losing weight.

REJECT THE "DIET"

- ◊ "Fad diets," while popular, are not supported by peer-reviewed literature.
- ◊ They distract providers and patients from implementing the simple solution of a whole-food, plant-based diet.
- ◊ Due to their temporary, restrictive nature, fad diets are difficult to implement as a lifestyle change and rarely promote weight maintenance in the long term.
- ◊ "Detox" diets and liquid-based "cleanses" may lead to initial weight loss, but this loss likely represents water. Greatly restricted caloric intake may decrease metabolic rate, leading to weight gain back to baseline once the patient resumes his normal eating pattern.[49]

> While there is little evidence for fad diets, **intermitting fasting** may be beneficial in preventing chronic disease and increasing longevity.[50]
> For example, it may improve insulin sensitivity and glucose tolerance.
> Fasting has also been shown to delay tumor progression in mice.[51]

SUGAR-SWEETENED BEVERAGES (SSBS)

- ◊ Include soda/soft drinks, juice, lemonade and sweetened tea, **sports and energy drinks, and sugary coffee drinks.**
- ◊ Contribute significantly to weight gain and obesity.
- ◊ In two studies, BMI decreased by an average of 0.25 kg/m^2 per day for every serving of SSB that was replaced by water.[52]
- ◊ Sports drinks such as Gatorade often contain excess sugar, and are unnecessary for most people with less than strenuous activity level.[53]

Did you know?

Several cities now have taxes on soda. Berkeley, California was the first US city to pass the tax and saw a 21% decrease in soda consumption.[54]

Sweetened coffee drinks can be loaded with sugar. A Starbucks Frappuccino (16oz) contains 50g-70g of sugar!

HEALTHY SNACKING

Snacks can be beneficial, helping to tame hunger during a long workday and prevent the end-of-the-day food binge. They can also help stabilize mood. However, snacking in the US is associated with weight gain, as most processed snacks are high in fat and salt and low in nutrients. Here are some tips for healthy snacking –

◊ Snack in the early morning (between breakfast and lunch) and limit snacks late at night.
◊ Try to stop eating 12 hours before you eat breakfast (i.e., stop eating at 8pm if you eat breakfast at 8am).
◊ Make at least one snack per day a fruit or vegetable. Consider pairing with a protein (for example, an organic apple with nut butter).
◊ Plan your snacks ahead of time and bring them with you. Avoid unplanned snacks and the vending machine.
◊ Ask yourself before a snack – Am I hungry? Or just thirsty? Can I wait until my next meal? Am I just bored, frustrated, or anxious? *What is it that I really seek?*

Snack option: Granola bars

◊ If purchasing pre-made granola bars, look for –
  o Sugar: **less than 6g**
  o Protein: at least 2g
  o Fiber: at least 2g
◊ Healthy options – Trader Joe's Rolled Oats and Peanut Butter Fiberful Granola Bars; Kashi chewy granola bars
◊ Be aware of **high sugar content** in energy and protein bars such as Clif bars.
◊ Make your own granola bars (recipe below).

Recipe: Homemade granola bars (no baking required!)

Makes about 12 bars

Ingredients
- 3 cups rolled oats
- 1 cup nuts of choice (pumpkin seeds, chopped almonds, or peanuts), raw or toasted
- ½ cup dried cranberries or raisins, chopped
- 1 cup peanut butter (use peanut butter powder and water for a lower-calorie option)
- ½ cup honey or brown rice syrup
- ¼ teaspoon sea salt
- 1 tablespoon chia seeds (optional)

Instructions
- Line a baking dish (such as a shallow 13x9 or 8-inch square pan) with aluminum foil or plastic wrap.
- Mix oats, nuts, cranberries/raisins, and chia seeds (if using) in large bowl.
- In a smaller bowl, whisk together nut butter, honey or brown rice syrup, and salt (warm slightly on the stove if not soft).
- Pour wet mixture into bowl with oats and mix well (with clean hands!) until well combined. Mixture should be sticky; if not, add more honey or plant-based milk such as unsweetened almond milk.
- Place mixture in lined baking dish and press down until flat. Cover with the foil or plastic wrap and place in refrigerator for at least 3 hours.
- Remove and cut into bars. To keep longer, wrap each bar in plastic wrap.

INTUITIVE EATING

Intuitive eating means listening to your senses of hunger and satiety to guide how often and how much you eat. It allows you to be aware of your inner mental state while eating or thinking of eating.

◊ Principles and tips[55] –
  o Drink a full glass of water when you feel hungry, as thirst can mimic hunger.
  o Sit down for every meal.
  o Eliminate distractions when eating snacks and meals. Stop working, hide your phone, turn off the TV, and avoid browsing social media.
  o Take a few deep breaths before eating.
  o Eat slowly, chewing and tasting your food. Put down your fork in between every bite.
  o Stop eating when you are satisfied and not quite "full." Wait 15 minutes before eating more, observing for the sensation of fullness.
  o Practice setting a timer for 30 minutes and try to take the whole time to consume your meal.

◊ The STOP mnemonic provides a mindfulness meditation for eating[56] –
  o Savor – First bite: When you take your first bite, notice the tastes developing. Focus fully on eating. Chew slowly and wait to swallow until the food is fully chewed.
  o Travel – Second bite: Focus on the source of the food – think about the place (farm, ocean, or garden) from which it came.
  o Observe – Third bite: Observe yourself as you eat. Notice how your hands, teeth, tongue, and body move. When you swallow, follow the food down to your stomach.
  o Pause – Fourth bite: Take an extra pause before putting the food into your mouth. Then pause again in the middle of chewing, and again after swallowing and before your next bite.

◊ Intuitive eating aims to create a healthy relationship with food and therefore discourages dieting and calorie counting. However, for those trying to lose weight, initial calorie counting may be beneficial to avoid underestimating caloric intake.[57]

> **"Emotional eating"** describes the tendency to choose the instant gratification of comfort foods when we are feeling frustrated, sad, or angry.
>
> Emotions also work the other way – **happy moods may make us choose better foods.** A study conducted at the University of Delaware examined the effects of positivity on eating. Reading a positive article caused participants to choose a healthier food over a "comfort food" higher in calories. In a separate study, reading a negative article caused participants to choose comfort foods.[58]

Obesity – Bottom Line

- Eat a balanced diet of whole, unprocessed foods – rich in vegetables, fruits, and whole grains, with protein from lean and plant sources.
- Emphasize *energy dilute* foods (vegetables, fruits, and complex carbs).
- Practice intuitive eating to help control portion sizes and mindless eating.
- Replace simple sugars and refined carbohydrates with complex carbohydrates such as whole grains. Avoid processed snacks and sugar-sweetened beverages.
- Restrict total fat somewhat, incorporating healthy fats (nuts, seeds, oils) with careful portion sizes.
- Combine with exercise, stress reduction, and good sleep habits for the most health benefit.

DIABETES

The incidence of Type 2 diabetes has increased with the obesity epidemic in America, and excess weight is the most significant modifiable risk factor.

- Type 2 diabetes arises from insulin resistance, which leads to decreased glucose uptake in skeletal muscle, liver, and adipose tissue. When increased insulin requirements lead to pancreatic beta cell "fatigue," overt diabetes develops.
- Genetic disposition is not required for the development of diabetes. However, beta cell fatigue develops more rapidly in patients who are genetically predisposed.
- **Diabetes is preventable with modest weight loss** (2-4kg), shown in several studies.[59]
- In a well-designed randomized controlled trial, **lifestyle intervention of diet and exercise, with modest weight loss (5-7%), reduced the incidence of Type 2 diabetes in pre-diabetics by 58%**, compared with standard of care metformin (30%).[60]
- Plant-based diets that are associated with lower diabetes risk include: the Mediterranean diet, the DASH diet for hypertension, and vegetarianism/veganism.
- Complex carbs such as whole grains (high in fiber and low in glycemic load) are associated with reduced diabetes risk.
- Fiber helps maintain glycemic control by decreasing the glycemic impact of meals. High intake of soluble fiber (50g/day) has been shown to improve glycemic control and lipid levels in diabetics.[61]
- Substituting healthy unsaturated fats for unhealthy saturated and trans-fats improves glycemic control and helps prevent diabetes.[62,63]
- Fructose, the sugar found in whole fruit and honey, has a slow rate of digestion and absorption. It is healthy for diabetics, unless consumed in excess (>10% of daily calories).[64]
- Artificial sweeteners have not been shown to increase appetite or encourage overeating. Nor have they been proven to cause cancer.[65] However, diabetics benefit from reducing all sweeteners.
- Daily consumption of cinnamon by Type 2 diabetics may help improve glycemic control through insulin sensitizing effects.[18]

> Fructose
> (in whole fruit and honey)
> is preferred over refined sugar for diabetics.

Diabetes – Bottom Line

- Even modest (10%) weight loss is beneficial.
- Restrict refined grains, processed snacks and sugar sweetened beverages.
- Replace simple sugars and refined carbs with complex carbs.
- Gradually increase fiber in the diet with whole grains, vegetables, and whole fruits.
- Whole fruit is healthy (unless in excess causing weight gain). Eat 3-4 servings a day.
- Substitute healthy (PUFA and MUFA) fats for unhealthy fats from processed and fast foods.
- Decrease use of all sweeteners.

CARDIOVASCULAR DISEASE

"The present cardiovascular medicine approach can neither cure the disease nor end the epidemic and is financially unsustainable." – Caldwell B. Esselstyn, MD[6]

Heart disease is the number-one cause of death in the US.[66] Plant-based nutrition can prevent cardiovascular disease.[67,68] A highly motivated patient can achieve the lipid-lowering effect of a statin simply by following a plant-based diet.[69] Diet is especially important in patients who cannot tolerate the side effects of statins, namely myalgia.

- Obesity is a cardiovascular disease risk factor, therefore weight loss is beneficial. Central/abdominal obesity is particularly worrisome for cardiovascular health.
- Vegetarians and vegans have low cardiovascular mortality and all-cause mortality.
- In a recent study, 7 days of a plant-based, low-fat diet lowered cholesterol by 22mg/dL, systolic blood pressure by 8mmHg, and 10-year risk of cardiovascular events to less than 7.5%. The effect was independent of weight loss.[70]
- Another study showed improvement and even reversal of coronary artery disease in patients who followed a plant-based, vegan diet for an average of 3.7 years.[6] Whole grains, legumes, fruits and vegetables composed most of the diet, with avoidance of meat, dairy, oils, and processed foods. **Recurrence of cardiovascular events was 0.6% in adherent patients and 62% in non-adherent patients.**

> A single egg yolk exceeds the daily recommended intake of cholesterol, and some individuals may experience a rise in LDL cholesterol with regular egg consumption. Those at risk for cardiovascular disease may benefit from eating less eggs.[71]

> Fiber is associated with lower lipid levels. Soluble fiber (found in foods such as **oatmeal**) lowers LDL cholesterol by binding bile acids.

The role of dietary fat

Certain fats are associated with elevated LDL cholesterol.

- ◊ Saturated fat from meats, processed foods, and fast food is associated with elevated LDL.[72] Saturated fat from dairy is *not* associated with increased cardiovascular risk.
- ◊ Other components of meat may also affect cardiovascular health – for example, red meat contains heme iron and processed meat contains preservatives.
- ◊ Of all fats, trans-fats contribute most to LDL and atherosclerosis.
- ◊ The traditional Mediterranean diet emphasizes monounsaturated and polyunsaturated fats and is associated with improved cardiovascular health.[73] The PREDIMED trial in 2013 showed that the Mediterranean diet, especially olive oil and mixed nut supplementation, reduced rates of cardiovascular events and mortality (up to a 30% relative risk reduction in patients with high CV risk). The strongest evidence was for reduction in cerebrovascular events.[74]

> Trans-fat is found in cookies and cakes, frozen biscuits, breakfast sandwiches, donuts, microwave popcorn, and fried fast food.

> **Did you know?**
>
> In 2015 the FDA ordered that all processed food companies eliminate partially hydrogenated oils (trans-fats) within three years.[75]

Nuts, especially **walnuts**, can **decrease triglycerides** and are associated with heart health.[76] They contain protein, fiber, and omega-3 fatty acids in varying amounts. Choose unroasted, unsalted nuts with no added sugar.

- Least healthy - all nuts roasted in partially hydrogenated oils
- Less healthy - macadamia nuts, hazelnuts, pine nuts, cashews
    - Contain the most calories per ounce and the least protein and fiber
- Somewhat healthy - pecans, pistachios
    - High caloric content per ounce, with less protein and fiber
    - Pecans contain a high number of antioxidants (similar to walnuts)
- Healthy - peanuts, almonds
    - Peanuts are high in protein and contain folate and vitamin E
    - Almonds are high in fiber and have the most calcium of all nuts
- Healthiest – walnuts *(Note: recommended portion size is just 2 walnuts!)*
    - With high amounts of omega-3 fatty acids and antioxidants, they may even be protective against cancer. In one study the blood of subjects consuming walnuts suppressed breast cancer proliferation in vitro.[77]

Heart disease – Bottom Line

- Avoid processed and fast foods to lower saturated and trans-fat intake.
- Limit red meat, factory-farmed and processed meat to avoid unhealthy saturated fat and other harmful ingredients.
- Reduce use of creamy sauces and dressings with hidden saturated and trans-fat content.
- Cook with olive oil instead of butter.
- Choose healthy unsaturated fats like nuts, olives, avocados, and olive oil.
- Consume generous amounts of fruits and vegetables for antioxidants and fiber.
- Consume healthy nuts (be aware of portion sizes).

HYPERTENSION

Dietary changes can effectively treat Stage I hypertension (140-160).[78]

- Central obesity and insulin resistance independently predict hypertension.[79] Modest weight loss can help lower blood pressure.
- Meat consumption is associated with higher blood pressure.[80]
- The Dietary Approaches to Stop Hypertension (DASH) diet, a plant-based diet high in vegetables, fruits, and whole grains and restricting saturated and trans-fats, can lower blood pressure 6-11 mmHg.[78]
- Adding salt restriction reduces BP even further.[81]
- About 50% of hypertensives are salt-sensitive, meaning that their blood pressure responds to salt intake. African Americans are more prone to salt sensitivity.[82]
- Excess alcohol may be a potential cause of resistant hypertension. Recommendations for moderate alcohol intake are up to 1 drink per day for women, and up to 2 drinks per day for men.[83]

> The vast majority of adults consume above the American Heart Association's recommended daily salt intake.

> **Does caffeine cause high blood pressure?**
>
> In studies, caffeine has not been shown to cause high blood pressure nor cardiac arrhythmias such as atrial fibrillation.[1]

Hypertension – Bottom Line

- Limit meat, especially red and processed meat.
- Use salt sparingly. If needed, add salt as food is consumed, rather than in the cooking process.
- Read food labels for hidden salt content in processed foods and canned goods.
- Avoid excess alcohol intake.
- Consume a diet rich in vegetables, fruits, and whole grains.

CANCER

Although cancer is a highly unpredictable disease, maintaining a healthy weight and eating a whole-food, plant-based diet can reduce risk of some cancers. For example, vegetarians have a lower risk of colorectal cancer, and pesco-vegetarians (who consume fish but not other meat) have an even lower risk – an estimated 43% lower.[84]

◊ Obesity is associated with increased cancer risk. A 34-pound weight gain may increase cancer risk by 10% (for colon, gallbladder, kidney, and liver cancers).[85] Mechanisms may involve hormones and inflammation due to adipose tissue.

Diet and colon cancer

◊ Colorectal cancer risk is associated with obesity and the high-fat, processed diet in the US.[86]
◊ **Red meat and processed meat have been strongly associated with risk of colon cancer.**[87] In 30 prospective studies, daily consumption of 50g (2oz) of processed meat was associated with a 20% increase in risk of colorectal cancer. Increased risk may be due to heterocyclic amines (carcinogens) in cured meats and heme iron in red meat.[88]
◊ Lean meats (fish, skinless poultry) are not associated with cancer. Grass-fed beef is associated with lower cancer risk than factory-farmed beef, which contains pesticides.
◊ High fiber intake is associated with decreased risk of colorectal cancer. Good gut bacteria ferment fiber to produce acids, creating a lower stool pH that is protective.[89]

Processed meat is meat that has been smoked, charred, cured, or otherwise processed. It includes bacon, sausage, deli meat, hot dogs, and fast food patties.

What about soy?

Soy intake appears to be safe and has not been shown to contribute to cancer risk in human trials. Soy intake has **not** been definitively linked to breast cancer.[1]

Eastern populations who consume more unprocessed soy (and less processed meat) have lower rates of cancer. Try to eat unprocessed and fermented soy (miso, tofu, tempeh, edamame), rather than processed soy (cereals, energy bars, packaged soy crumbles).

ANTIOXIDANTS

- ◊ Antioxidants are micronutrients that protect the body against oxidation, the process by which oxygen radicals damage the cells of the body.
- ◊ They include Vitamins C and E, as well as anthocyanins (found in berries), catechins (found in green tea), flavonoids (found in kale and apples), resveratrol (found in red wine and grapes), and carotenoids (found in some vegetables).
- ◊ Intake of antioxidants in food – but not vitamins/supplements – is associated with lower cancer risk, as well as lower risk of heart disease and stroke.
- ◊ One 2012 study showed that increasing intake of green leafy vegetables to one serving per day may cut risk of Non-Hodgkin Lymphoma in half.[90]

Antioxidant-rich fruits and vegetables[91,92]

- ◊ Vegetables – cruciferous vegetables (broccoli, brussel sprouts, cauliflower), dark leafy greens, eggplant, beets, red pepper
- ◊ Fruits – cranberries, apples, red grapes, strawberries, lemons, peaches

Cancer – Bottom Line

- Maintaining a healthy weight, along with exercise and avoiding smoke exposure, can help prevent many types of cancer.
- Make whole grains, cruciferous vegetables, and legumes the main part of a meal.
- Avoid intake of red and processed meat entirely or consume as a "treat". If you are a meat eater, try to eat it no more than two times per week (4 ounce portions), and choose lean meats (fish/chicken or turkey), preferably organic.
- Incorporate antioxidant-rich fruits and vegetables into every meal.

GASTROINTESTINAL DISEASE

Gluten sensitivity

◊ Celiac disease, or autoimmune gluten intolerance, affects approximately 1% of the US population.[93]
◊ "Non-celiac" gluten sensitivity remains a contested diagnosis. Unlike celiac disease, it does not involve gliadin-mediated mucosal inflammation.
◊ Non-celiac sensitivity to gluten-containing foods may actually represent an intolerance to FODMAPS (Fermentable Oligosaccharides, Disaccharides, Monosaccharides and Polyols), which also cause GI discomfort in patients with Irritable Bowel Syndrome.[94]

> Gluten is found in wheat and flour, rye, barley, cereals, pasta, crackers, and breadcrumbs, as well as in other foods such as beer, soups, sausages, and energy bars.[95] Gluten-free grains include rice, quinoa, buckwheat, gluten-free oats, and millet.

IRRITABLE BOWEL SYNDROME (IBS)

- ◊ IBS is classified as diarrhea-predominant or constipation-predominant.
- ◊ Patients with both types of IBS benefit from gradually increasing fiber intake.
- ◊ IBS symptoms may improve with a trial of a gluten-free diet. Patients may also try a diet low in FODMAPs, which are carbohydrate components that are difficult to digest.

High FODMAP foods (limit in IBS)[96]

- ◊ Garlic, onion
- ◊ Beans
- ◊ Cauliflower
- ◊ Apples
- ◊ Wheat and cereals
- ◊ Artificial sweeteners – xylitol, sorbitol

Low FODMAP foods (okay in IBS)

- ◊ Lettuce
- ◊ Zucchini
- ◊ Sweet potato
- ◊ Bananas, oranges, berries
- ◊ Quinoa, millet, brown rice
- ◊ Soy (tofu, tempeh)
- ◊ Eggs

The gut microbiome and probiotics

◊ The gut is populated by bacteria after birth and is influenced by diet in adulthood. The "good" gut bacteria defend against pathogenic bacteria such as *E.coli*.
◊ The gut microbiome also affects inflammatory states, skin conditions, and weight.[97]
◊ Probiotics may help replace good gut bacteria and prevent bacterial overgrowth that causes gas and bloating in IBS.
◊ The species *B. infantis, B. bifidum, and VSL#3* may be beneficial in IBS.[98]
◊ *Lactobacillus rhamnosus* and *Saccharomyces boulardii* have been shown to reduce the risk of antibiotic-associated colitis in pediatric patients.[99]

Probiotics vs Prebiotics

◊ **Probiotics** – active beneficial bacteria found in food and probiotic supplements. Found in fermented foods – yogurt, kimchi, tempeh, sauerkraut, kombucha, and pickled vegetables.

◊ **Prebiotics** – food components that feed the good gut bacteria, which ferment them to produce anti-inflammatory products. Found in plant foods with **fiber,** onions, raw garlic, and artichokes.

Gastrointestinal Disease – Bottom Line

- Patients with non-celiac gluten sensitivity and IBS may benefit from a gluten-free and/or low-FODMAP diet.
- Patients with IBS also benefit from gradually increasing fiber intake.
- Promote the growth of good gut bacteria by consuming probiotics and prebiotics.
- Consume probiotics in fermented foods (sauerkraut, yogurt) and/or in supplements.
- Consume prebiotics in fiber-containing foods and other unprocessed plant foods, such as garlic, asparagus, and artichokes.

NEUROLOGIC DISEASE

The brain is the command center for many vital processes in the body. Common conditions such as headache and cognitive impairment are affected by nutrition. In addition, the painful neuropathy associated with Type 2 diabetes may be preventable with diet.

When looking at the effect of malnutrition on the central nervous system, brain imaging can reveal abnormal appearance of the mamillary bodies, anterior thalamus, corpus callosum, and cerebellum. These lesions are similar to what has been long described in Wernicke encephalopathy and the malnutrition resulting from alcohol use.[100,101]

Headache

Obesity itself can exacerbate headaches, such as those seen in cases of weight-related Obstructive Sleep Apnea and Idiopathic Intracranial Hypertension. In addition, a subset of patients experience migraines that are triggered or improved by certain foods.

- ◊ Common food triggers for migraine are highly variable, but include red wine, chocolate, processed meats (especially hot dogs), and MSG (monosodium glutamate).[102]
    - o Processed meat contains nitrites, which produce vasodilation through nitric oxide.
    - o MSG may affect glutamate transmission in the brain.
    - o Red wine contains histamine and induces vascular headaches (migraines) in individuals who are deficient in the enzyme that metabolizes histamine.
    - o Individuals sensitive to histamine may also experience headaches with cheese, sausage, sauerkraut, tomatoes, tuna and other histamine-rich foods.
- ◊ Other headache triggers include caffeine withdrawal, caffeine excess, dehydration, and fasting or skipping meals.

◊ Keeping a headache diary of foods consumed before and during a headache may help to identify food triggers.
◊ A trial of an elimination diet may also be helpful – patients should remove one food item for a few weeks and observe for improvement.

> **Caffeine consumption** is another common cause of headache and disturbed sleep. Counsel patients on how much caffeine is in their favorite beverages[103] –
>
> ◊ Coffee (8oz) – 95-200mg
> ◊ Energy drink (8-16oz) – 50-200mg
> ◊ Espresso (2oz) – 45-75mg
> ◊ Black tea (8oz) – 15-70mg
> ◊ Green tea (8oz) – 24-45mg – ***also rich in antioxidants!***
> ◊ Caffeinated soft drink (12oz) – 20-50mg
> ◊ Iced/sweet tea (8oz) – 10-45mg
> ◊ Square of dark chocolate – 40-75mg

Dementia

◊ Certain vitamin and mineral deficiencies, such as Vitamin B deficiencies, can lead to cognitive difficulty.
◊ Besides frank vitamin deficiency, the strongest evidence for nutrition in preventing age-related cognitive decline is for fruit and vegetable intake.[1] Antioxidants in fruits and vegetables prevent against oxidative injury.
◊ Vitamin E is an antioxidant, and consumption in food may be protective in cognitive health. However, there is no convincing evidence for Vitamin E supplementation in the prevention or treatment of Alzheimer dementia.
◊ Unsaturated fatty acids, especially PUFAs (olive, nuts, and seeds) may be beneficial in preventing cognitive decline.[104]

- Fish consumption is of uncertain benefit for cognitive health.
    - Fish contains omega-3 fatty acids, specifically DHA, that are neuroprotective.[105]
    - Recent meta-analyses have shown inconclusive evidence for the effect of fish on cognitive function.[106]
    - Omega-3 supplementation with fish oil has not consistently demonstrated cognitive benefit in studies and more research is needed. Supplementation is unlikely to be harmful.
- Obesity is associated with increased risk of cognitive decline, therefore maintaining a healthy weight – along with exercising and good sleep habits – may be beneficial.

Neurologic Disease – Bottom Line

- Food triggers are variable, and headache patients may benefit from keeping a food diary followed by an elimination diet.
- Common headache triggers include red wine, processed meat, and caffeine withdrawal.
- Antioxidant intake in fruits and vegetables over a lifetime may help prevent cognitive decline, when combined with exercise and sleep.
- Other supplements such as Vitamin E and fish oil have not been shown to prevent dementia.

PART FOUR: PLANT-BASED RECIPES

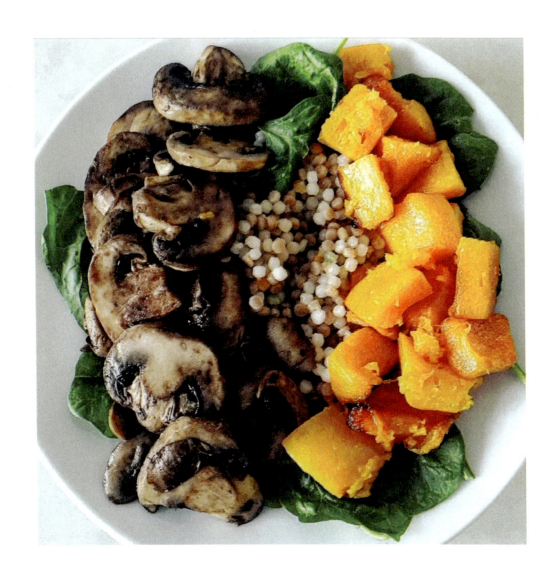

BREAKFAST

Overnight oats

- ◊ Prep time: overnight (or at least 8 hours)
- ◊ Makes 2-3 servings
- ◊ Ingredients
    - 1 ½ cup old-fashioned rolled oats
    - 1 ½ cup plant-based milk (try almond or hemp milk)
    - ½ cup water
    - 2 tablespoons chia seeds (optional)
    - 1 tablespoon honey or maple syrup
    - 1 teaspoon cinnamon
    - 1 teaspoon vanilla extract
    - Optional toppings: fresh or frozen fruit, nuts (almonds, walnuts), or nut butter
- ◊ Instructions
    - Place all ingredients except toppings into a medium bowl or large mason jar. Mix well. Seal shut and place in refrigerator overnight.
    - In the morning, mix again and add toppings of choice (fresh fruit, nuts, spoonful of nut butter).
    - Store in refrigerator up to 3-4 days.

Homemade granola

- ◊ Makes 8-10 servings
- ◊ Ingredients
    - Coconut oil or canola oil
    - 3 cups rolled oats
    - ½ cup raw walnuts, chopped
    - ½ cup raw almonds, chopped
    - ½ cup raw peanuts or pumpkin seeds
    - ½ cup raisins or cranberries
    - ½ cup maple syrup or honey
    - ¼ teaspoon salt
    - ¼ teaspoon cinnamon
    - Optional: ½ cup popped amaranth or ½ cup toasted buckwheat
- ◊ Instructions
    - Preheat oven to 325 degrees F. Lightly coat a large baking sheet with oil (or spray with cooking spray).
    - In a medium bowl combine oats, nuts, maple syrup, salt, cinnamon, and raisins/cranberries if using.
    - Spread mixture in one even layer onto baking sheet and bake until golden brown, checking and turning every 10 minutes to ensure it does not burn, for about 25 minutes.
    - Optional: add popped amaranth or toasted buckwheat to baked granola.
    - Let cool completely before storing in an airtight container.

Vegan banana walnut pancakes

- Makes about 12 pancakes
- Ingredients
    - 1 cup whole wheat flour
    - 1 cup almond, coconut, or garbanzo flour
    - 1 tablespoon baking powder
    - ½ teaspoon salt
    - 1 teaspoon cinnamon
    - 1 ½ tablespoons maple syrup
    - 2 cups plant-based milk (try unsweetened almond milk)
    - 1 teaspoon apple cider vinegar
    - 2 tablespoons coconut oil, melted
    - 1 teaspoon vanilla extract
    - 1 ripe banana, mashed
    - 1/3 cup raw walnuts, chopped
- Instructions
    - In a large bowl, whisk together both types of flour, baking powder, salt, and cinnamon.
    - In a medium bowl, combine plant-based milk and apple cider vinegar and whisk until frothy. Stir in coconut oil, vanilla, and maple syrup.
    - Add wet to dry mixture and stir until smooth. Add mashed banana and walnuts. Add more plant-based milk as needed so that batter is not too thick.
    - Heat skillet or griddle over medium-high heat and coat lightly with coconut oil. When skillet is hot, pour on pancake batter (about ¼ to 1/3 cup). Flip the pancake when you see bubbles forming on one side.
    - Repeat to use all of batter.
    - Serve with maple syrup, almond butter, or fresh fruit.

Zucchini muffins

- Serves: 12
- Ingredients
    - 2 cups whole wheat flour or almond flour
    - 1 cup rolled oats
    - 1 tablespoon ground cinnamon
    - 1 teaspoon baking soda
    - ½ teaspoon salt
    - 2 eggs
    - 1 medium zucchini, grated and water squeezed out (about 1 cup)
    - 1/3 cup coconut oil, melted
    - ½ cup maple syrup or honey
    - 1 teaspoon vanilla extract
    - ½ cup walnuts, chopped
    - ½ cup raisins or cranberries (optional)
    - 2 tablespoons ground flaxseed (optional)
- Instructions
    - Preheat oven to 350 degrees F. Coat a 12-muffin tin with coconut oil (or cooking spray).
    - In a large bowl, combine whole wheat or almond flour, rolled oats, cinnamon, baking soda, and salt.
    - In a medium bowl, add eggs and whisk. Add zucchini, carrots, coconut oil, maple syrup or honey, and vanilla.
    - Add wet to dry ingredients. Fold in walnuts, raisins/cranberries, and flaxseed if using.
    - If mixture is too dry, add ¼ cup unsweetened plant-based milk such as almond milk.
    - Spoon mixture into muffin tin, filling about ¾ of the way. Bake 25-30 minutes, until golden brown.

Tofu sweet potato bake

- Makes 4 servings
- Ingredients
    - 2 medium sweet potatoes, diced
    - 1 red bell pepper, diced
    - 1 (15.5oz) package firm or extra firm tofu, drained and diced (To drain tofu, remove from package and place between two cloths or paper towels, then place under a heavy item such as a book.)
    - 1 yellow or white onion, diced
    - 3 tablespoons olive oil or coconut oil
    - 1 teaspoon sea salt, plus more to taste
    - ¼ teaspoon black pepper, plus more to taste
    - ½ teaspoon turmeric or cumin
    - ½ teaspoon dried oregano
    - ¼ cup pumpkin seeds
- Instructions
    - Preheat oven to 400 degrees F.
    - Toast pumpkin seeds in oven or in a sauté pan until just browned.
    - In a large bowl, combine sweet potatoes, bell pepper, tofu, and onions. Add olive oil, salt, pepper, turmeric or cumin, and oregano, and mix together. Add toasted pumpkin seeds.
    - Spread mixture in a 9 x 13 in (3.5L) baking dish and bake for 30-45 minutes. Potatoes should be soft and tofu just browned.
    - Serve warm with eggs or in tortillas with avocado and salsa.

Green smoothie

Makes about 4 servings

Ingredients
- 1 banana, peeled and frozen
- ½ cup strawberries or mango
- 1 cup fresh spinach leaves
- 1 cup unsweetened plant-based milk (such as almond milk)
- Optional: 1 teaspoon vanilla extract, 1 spoonful of avocado, 1 tablespoon fresh mint or ginger

Instructions
Place all ingredients in blender and puree until creamy.

Muesli

Muesli is a traditional breakfast cereal that combines oats, nuts and seeds, and fruit. Unlike granola, it does not require baking and contains no added sugar or oil.

Makes 4 servings

Ingredients
- 2 cups rolled oats, uncooked or toasted over low heat
- ¼ cup chopped dates, raisins, or cranberries
- ¼ cup walnuts or almonds, chopped
- ¼ cup pumpkin seeds
- ½ teaspoon cinnamon
- 3 ½ cups unsweetened plant-based milk such as almond milk
- ½ cup plain Greek yogurt (optional)
- 2 tablespoons honey if desired

Instructions
Mix all ingredients except milk and yogurt in a large bowl. Eat for breakfast with plant-based milk or yogurt. Add fresh fruit or honey for sweetness.
You can also eat muesli like oatmeal. To make overnight muesli, stir all ingredients including milk (and yogurt if using) in a large bowl. Cover and refrigerate overnight. In morning, add a touch more milk if desired and stir again. Add honey or fresh fruit for sweetness.

LUNCH

Marinated tofu and Bok choy salad

- ◊ Makes 2-3 servings
- ◊ Prep time: overnight; cook time: 1 hour
- ◊ Ingredients – Marinated tofu
    - o 1 (16 ounce) package firm or extra-firm tofu
    - o 3 tablespoons soy sauce or liquid amino's
    - o 1 garlic clove, minced
    - o 1 tablespoon fresh grated ginger, (or ½ teaspoon ground ginger)
    - o 1 tablespoon coconut oil or olive oil, plus more for pan
    - o 1 tablespoon rice wine vinegar (optional)
    - o 1 teaspoon honey or maple syrup
    - o 1 teaspoon cumin or turmeric
- ◊ Instructions – Marinated tofu
    - o Drain tofu (remove from package, and place between two cloths or paper towels, then place under a heavy item such as a book). Cut into 1 inch cubes.
    - o Mix all other ingredients together.
    - o Pour marinade over tofu and gently coat. Cover bowl and refrigerate overnight.
    - o Preheat oven to 350 degrees F. Lightly grease baking sheet with olive oil or coconut oil.
    - o Arrange marinated tofu in single layer on sheet.
    - o Bake at 350 degrees for 35-40 minutes, flipping tofu about every 15 minutes, until golden brown and crispy.
- ◊ Ingredients – Bok choy salad
    - o 2 heads Bok choy, leaves and white parts chopped in small pieces
    - o 2 cups kale, chopped in small pieces
    - o 3 green onions, green and some of white parts chopped
    - o ½ cup slivered almonds
    - o ¼ cup soy sauce or liquid amino's
    - o ¼ cup olive oil
    - o ¼ cup rice vinegar or white vinegar
    - o 1 tablespoon honey
    - o 1 tablespoon squeeze lemon or lime
- ◊ Instructions – Bok choy salad
    - o Combine Bok choy, kale, green onions, and almonds in large bowl.
    - o To make dressing – combine soy sauce, olive oil, vinegar, honey, and lemon/lime juice and whisk with fork to combine.
    - o Pour dressing onto salad, massaging kale in dressing to soften.
    - o Serve as a side dish or topped with marinated tofu.

Roasted chickpea snack

- Serves: 2-3
- Ingredients
    - 1 can (15oz) chickpeas (garbanzo beans)
    - 2 teaspoons olive oil
    - ½ teaspoon salt
    - ½ teaspoon cumin
    - ½ teaspoon chili powder
    - ½ teaspoon curry powder (optional)
- Instructions
    - Preheat oven to 400 degrees F.
    - Drain chickpeas, rinse, and pat dry. (Peel off their outer layer to make them crispier after baking.) Add to large bowl.
    - In a small bowl, mix spices and olive oil together.
    - Add marinade to large bowl with chickpeas and mix to combine.
    - Lay flat in a single layer on a baking sheet and bake for 35-45 minutes, turning with spatula every 15 minutes.
- *Eat alone as a snack, or toss in a salad with avocado and optional feta cheese.*

Burrito bowl

- Makes 4 servings
- Ingredients
    - 1 cup quinoa or brown rice
    - 1 tablespoon olive oil or coconut oil
    - ¼ cup onion, diced
    - 1 bell pepper (any color), sliced into ¼ inch strips
    - 1 clove garlic, minced
    - 2 cans (15oz) black beans or pinto beans, drained and rinsed
    - ¼ teaspoon fresh cilantro, chopped
    - ¼ teaspoon chili powder
    - ¼ teaspoon cumin
    - ¼ cup squeezed lime juice
    - ½ cup diced tomato
    - ½ cup corn
    - Salt
    - Optional ingredients
        - Grated natural cheese, salsa, avocado or homemade guacamole
        - Romaine lettuce, chopped
- Instructions
    - Cook quinoa or brown rice in saucepan with 2 cups of water (if using quinoa, rinse and drain first). Bring to a boil, then reduce heat to a low simmer. Cover pot and simmer for 20 minutes until fluffy and water is absorbed.
    - Meanwhile, sauté onion and bell peppers in 1 tablespoon olive oil, stirring every 1-2 minutes, until browned, about 5-10 minutes. Add garlic and saute 1-2 minutes longer.
    - Add beans to pot with onions and peppers. Add ½ cup water, 2 tablespoons fresh cilantro, chili powder, and cumin. Bring to a boil, then reduce to medium low heat and simmer 15 minutes until liquid mostly absorbed. Stir in 2 tablespoons fresh lime juice. Add salt to taste.
    - Remove cooked quinoa or rice from heat and fluff with fork. Remove from heat and fluff with a fork. Mix in 2 tablespoons fresh cilantro, remaining fresh lime juice, and pinch of salt.
    - Assemble bowl with quinoa/rice and beans. Add diced tomato, corn, and fresh cilantro, as well as optional shredded lettuce, salsa, avocado/guacamole, and cheese.

Quinoa with roasted veggies

- Makes 6 servings
- Ingredients
    - 1 summer (yellow) squash, sliced into half moons
    - 1 medium zucchini, diced
    - 2 bell peppers (red, yellow, or orange), diced
    - 1 red onion, diced
    - 2 cloves garlic, minced
    - 1 cup grape or cherry tomatoes, halved
    - 4 tablespoons olive oil
    - ½ teaspoon salt, plus more to taste
    - ¼ teaspoon black pepper
    - 1 ½ cups quinoa (or substitute bulgur)
    - 3 cups low-sodium vegetable broth
    - 3 tablespoons balsamic vinegar
    - 1 teaspoon Dijon mustard
    - ¼ cups fresh parsley, chopped
    - ¼ cups fresh basil, chopped
    - 2 green onions, sliced (optional)
- Instructions
    - Preheat oven to 425 degrees F.
    - Place squash, zucchini, bell pepper, onion, and garlic on a baking sheet. Lightly coat with 2 tablespoons olive oil and season with salt and pepper. Place in oven and roast until vegetables are slightly toasted on edges, about 35-40 minutes.
    - Meanwhile, cook quinoa in saucepan. Bring vegetable broth to a bowl, add quinoa, and simmer covered for 15 minutes until broth is absorbed. Fluff with fork and season with salt to taste.
    - Add cooked quinoa and roasted vegetables in large bowl.
    - In small bowl, whisk 3 tablespoons olive oil with balsamic vinegar and Dijon mustard. Pour dressing over quinoa and vegetable mixture. Add parsley, basil, and green onion if using. Mix to combine.
    - Serve warm.

Baked Falafel with avocado sauce

- Makes about 10-12 falafel
- Ingredients – Falafel
    - 2 cloves garlic or ¼ teaspoon garlic powder
    - ¼ teaspoon onion powder
    - ½ cup fresh parsley or cilantro, leaves removed from stems
    - 2 cans (15oz) chickpeas, drained and rinsed
    - ¼ cup whole wheat flour or rolled oats ground into flour
    - 1 teaspoon cumin
    - 1 teaspoon coriander
    - ½ teaspoon turmeric
    - ¾ teaspoon salt
    - ¼ teaspoon black pepper
    - 1 tablespoon lemon juice
    - 2 tablespoons olive oil
    - 1 tablespoon tahini or peanut butter (optional)
- Ingredients – Avocado sauce
    - 1 avocado
    - 2 tablespoons olive oil
    - 2 tablespoons plain nonfat Greek yogurt
    - 1 tablespoon lemon juice
    - 2 tablespoons warm water
    - ¼ cup sunflower seeds
- Instructions – Baked falafel
    - Preheat oven to 375 degrees F.
    - Coat a large baking sheet with 1 tablespoon of olive oil.
    - Place garlic or garlic powder, onion powder, and parsley or cilantro in food processor until chopped. Add chickpeas, flour, cumin, coriander, salt, pepper, and lemon juice and pulse until smooth.
    - Roll mixture into about 12-15 balls and placed onto oiled baking sheet. Brush lightly with 1 tablespoon olive oil.
    - Bake for 25-30 minutes until just browned.
- Instructions – Avocado sauce
    - Combine avocado, yogurt, lemon, sunflower seeds, and warm water in food processor. Process until smooth. Add more water if sauce is too thick. Add salt to taste.
- Serve falafel topped with avocado sauce on a salad or with diced cucumbers and tomato in a pita.

DINNER

Lentil stuffed sweet potatoes

- ◊ Makes 4 servings
- ◊ Ingredients
    - o 4 medium sweet potatoes
    - o 1 tablespoon coconut oil or olive oil
    - o ½ medium white onion (about 3/4 cup), finely chopped
    - o 1 clove garlic, finely chopped
    - o 1 tablespoon curry powder
    - o ½ teaspoon turmeric
    - o 1 cup brown or green lentils
    - o 3 cups water
    - o ½ cup light coconut milk
    - o ½ teaspoon salt
    - o ¼ teaspoon black pepper
    - o ½ teaspoon apple cider vinegar
    - o 1 bunch fresh spinach
    - o ¼ cup plain Greek yogurt
    - o ½ cup fresh cilantro leaves
- ◊ Instructions
    - o Preheat oven to 400 degrees F.
    - o Pierce sweet potatoes with a knife and place on baking sheet. Bake until soft, about 45 minutes.
    - o Meanwhile, make the lentils. Heat the oil in a medium saucepan over medium heat. Add the onion and cook until softened and slightly brown, about 2-3 minutes. Add the garlic, curry powder, and turmeric and cook another minute. Add the lentils and water and bring to a boil. Reduce heat and simmer for 30 minutes until water is mostly absorbed.
    - o Stir in the coconut milk, salt, pepper, and apple cider vinegar and simmer another 5 minutes. Add fresh spinach and simmer 5 minutes more, until lentils are fully cooked and spinach is wilted.
    - o Cut a slit in the sweet potatoes and open them lengthwise. Soften the inside with a fork before spooning the lentils on top.
    - o Garnish with a spoonful of Greek yogurt and fresh cilantro.

White hominy chili

- Makes 6 servings
- Ingredients
    - 1 tablespoon olive oil
    - 1 medium onion, diced
    - 2 stalks celery, diced
    - 3 medium poblano peppers, seeded and finely diced
    - 1 clove garlic, minced
    - 1 teaspoon ground cumin
    - ½ teaspoon ground coriander
    - ¼ teaspoon cayenne pepper, more to taste
    - 2 (15oz) cans low-sodium white beans, drained and rinsed
    - 4 cups low-sodium vegetable broth
    - ¾ teaspoon dried oregano
    - 1 can (15oz) hominy, drained and rinsed
    - Salt
    - ¼ cup nonfat plain Greek yogurt
    - ½ cup fresh cilantro, chopped
    - 1 lime
- Instructions
    - Heat the oil in a large pot over medium heat.
    - Add the onion, celery, poblanos, and cook, stirring occasionally, until the vegetables are soft, about 5-7 minutes. Add the garlic, cumin, coriander, and cayenne and cook, stirring, about 30 seconds.
    - Add the beans, broth, and oregano. Cover partially and cook, stirring occasionally, for 25 minutes.
    - Add the hominy and salt and cook for 10 minutes longer. Ladle into bowls and top each serving with 1 tablespoon of Greek yogurt, fresh cilantro, and a squeeze of lime.

Butternut squash and pea risotto

Makes 4 servings

- Ingredients
    - 2 tablespoons olive oil
    - 1 onion, finely chopped
    - 2 cloves garlic, finely chopped
    - 1 ½ tablespoons fresh sage, or 1 teaspoon dried sage
    - 1 cup pearled barley
    - 1 (32oz) container vegetable broth
    - Salt and pepper
    - 1 small butternut squash, peeled and cut into bite-size pieces
    - 1 cup frozen peas
    - 1 cup natural grated parmesan cheese (optional) *Vegan option – substitute ¼ cup nutritional yeast, or 1 cup almond cheese
- Instructions
    - In a large saucepan or Dutch oven, heat the oil over medium heat. Add the onion and cook until softened, stirring, about 5 minutes.
    - Stir in the garlic and sage and cook for 1 minute. Add the vegetable broth and barley and stir. Add 1 teaspoon salt and ½ teaspoon pepper.
    - Bring to a boil, then reduce heat and simmer 15 minutes, covered.
    - Add the squash, cover the pot and cook until tender, 15 to 20 minutes. Stir in the peas and cheese or nutritional yeast. Cook, uncovered, for a few minutes until cheese is melted.

Build your own veggie burger

- ◊ Ingredients
  - o Base – 1 can (15oz) of **beans** + 1 cup of cooked **grains**
    - Beans – garbanzos, kidney beans, or black beans; drained and rinsed
    - Grains – brown rice, quinoa, or bulgur
    - Optional – use ½ can beans and add ½ \cup cooked sweet potato
  - o Add-ins – 1 ½ cups **vegetables** + ¼ cup of **nuts** (optional)
    - Vegetables – onions, carrots, mushrooms, broccoli, bell peppers; raw or sautéed in 1 tablespoon olive oil
    - Nuts – walnuts, sunflower seeds, almonds; raw or toasted; chopped or processed in food processor
  - o Binder – 1 cup of **flour**
    - Flour – Rolled oats processed in a food processor, garbanzo flour, brown rice flour, amaranth flour
    - Optional – use ½ cup flour and ½ cup whole grain breadcrumbs – *to make breadcrumbs, toast 2 slices of whole grain bread and process in food processor*
  - o Seasoning – **garlic** + **herbs and spices**
    - 2 cloves garlic, minced, raw or sautéed in 1 tablespoon olive oil – or ½ teaspoon garlic powder
    - Spices – cumin, turmeric, coriander
    - Herbs – rosemary, oregano (½ teaspoon dried or 1 tablespoon fresh), fresh cilantro or parsley (2 tablespoons fresh)
  - o Moistener
    - 2-3 tablespoons unsweetened plant-based milk (such as almond milk) or vegetable broth
    - Optional – one egg

- ◊ Instructions
    - Preheat oven to 350 degrees F. Lightly coat a baking sheet with olive oil.
    - Place beans in food processor and pulse until mostly smooth with a few chunks (if you don't have a food processor, you can mash them with a fork). Add cooked sweet potato if using and process to combine. Place in a large bowl and add cooked grain.
    - Finely chop vegetables in food processor or by hand. If sautéing, cook in 1 tablespoon of olive oil until soft. Add the vegetables to the bowl with beans and grain. Add raw or toasted nuts if using.
    - Add flour and optional breadcrumbs to bowl. Add garlic, herbs and spices and salt to taste. Knead mixture with hands until well combined. Add the almond milk or vegetable broth, or 1 egg if using, and combine until moist. Add 1 tablespoon olive oil.
    - Form patties about the size of your palm. Place on parchment paper on a baking sheet and place in refrigerator for at least an hour (this step is not necessary but helps burgers stick together better).
    - You can pat the surfaces of the burgers in more flour to form a crispy coating.
    - Bake on prepared baking sheet for 20-25 minutes, flipping every 10 minutes.
        - *You can also cook these in a sauté pan on the stove. Heat a teaspoon of olive oil on medium heat, place burger on pan, and cook for 5 minutes on each side.
    - Serve over a salad or on a whole-wheat bun with lettuce, tomato, and avocado.

Kale salad with quinoa and sweet potatoes + Dijon basil vinaigrette

Makes 4 servings

- Ingredients – Kale salad with quinoa and sweet potatoes
    - 2 medium sweet potatoes, diced into bite-size pieces
    - 2 tablespoons olive oil
    - Salt and pepper
    - 1 cup white quinoa
    - 1 ¾ cups vegetable broth
    - 1 bunch kale, stems removed and chopped into small pieces (about 3 cups)
    - ½ cup pumpkin seeds, raw or roasted and salted
- Ingredients – Dijon basil vinaigrette
    - ½ cup fresh basil leaves, finely chopped or processed in a food processor
    - ½ cup olive oil
    - Juice of ½ lemon (about ¼ cup)
    - 2 tablespoons apple cider vinegar
    - ½ tablespoon Dijon mustard
    - 1 teaspoon maple syrup or honey
    - ¼ teaspoon salt
    - Black pepper to taste
- Instructions
    - Preheat oven to 425 degrees F. Lightly coat a baking sheet with olive oil.
    - Place diced sweet potatoes in a medium bowl and toss with 2 tablespoons olive oil
    - Place on baking sheet in single layer. Bake for 20-30 minutes until soft and slightly brown.
    - Meanwhile, cook the quinoa. Rinse first in a sieve or strainer, then add to a medium saucepan with the vegetable broth. Bring to a boil, then reduce heat and simmer, partially covered, about 25 minutes, until quinoa absorbs all of broth. Fluff with a fork.
    - To make the vinaigrette - combine all of the ingredients in a small bowl and whisk to combine.
    - Place chopped kale in a large bowl or serving dish. Add the quinoa, sweet potatoes, and dressing. Massage the kale with your hands until it is slightly wilted.
    - If using raw pumpkin seeds, heat a skillet on low-medium heat and toast the pumpkin seeds for 3-5 minutes until fragrant and slightly browned. Add pumpkin seeds to the salad and toss.
    - Serve at room temperature.

Moroccan Cauliflower and Quinoa

- Serves: 6
- Ingredients
    - 1 large cauliflower head
    - 2 lemons
    - 1 tablespoon paprika
    - 2 teaspoons ground coriander
    - ½ teaspoon sea salt
    - 1 teaspoon black pepper
    - 2 tablespoon olive oil
    - 1 large onion, chopped
    - 3 garlic cloves, minced
    - 1 cup dried apricots, roughly chopped
    - 1 cup quinoa
    - 2 cups vegetable or bone broth
    - ½ cup sliced almonds
    - ½ cup cilantro, chopped
- Instructions
    - Separate cauliflower into 1 inch florets
    - Steam cauliflower in 1-2 cups water until tender, drain and set aside
    - Juice one of the lemons and thinly slice the other. Cut the slices into small pieces of lemon rind and set aside.
    - In a mixing bowl, combine the paprika, coriander, cumin, salt and pepper and stir to combine. Add the cauliflower and toss to coat.
    - In a large skillet with a lid over medium heat, heat the olive oil. Add the cauliflower, saute until slightly browned, stirring frequently, for 5 minutes. Add the cut up lemon pieces, onion, garlic and apricots. Cook, stirring frequently until the onion softens, 5 minutes. Add the quinoa and cook, stirring, for 3-4 minutes. Add the vegetable or bone broth and lemon juice. Raise the heat and bring to a boil. Cover the pan, lower the heat to medium low and cook covered for 20 minutes or until the liquid has been absorbed and the quinoa is tender. Remove from the heat and let sit, covered, for 5 minutes.
    - While the quinoa and cauliflower sits, toast the almond slices. In a small, dry skillet over medium heat, toast the almonds for a few minutes stirring often until they are browned and fragrant.
    - To serve, put the quinoa cauliflower mixture in a serving bowl, fluff gently with a fork and top with the toasted almonds and cilantro.

Potato and pepita enchiladas

- Makes about 8-10 enchiladas
- Ingredients
    - 1 bunch curly kale or Swiss chard, chopped into small pieces (remove stems at ends)
    - 1 tablespoon olive oil or coconut oil
    - 1 white onion, diced
    - ½ teaspoon salt
    - 2 medium sweet potatoes or red potatoes, diced
    - Salt
    - Black pepper
    - ½ teaspoon apple cider vinegar
    - ½ cup raw pumpkin seeds (pepitas)
    - 1 can (4 cups) red enchilada sauce
    - ¼ teaspoon coconut oil (optional)
    - 10-15 small corn or sprouted grain tortillas
    - Fresh cilantro leaves, for garnish
    - Optional – natural cheese of choice for garnish
- Instructions
    - Preheat oven to 350 degrees F.
    - In a large sauté pan, heat 1 tablespoon oil over medium heat. Add onions and cook until softened and slightly brown, about 5 minutes. Add kale or swiss chard and ¼ cup of water. Sprinkle with salt. Cover and cook, about 10 minutes, until wilted. Remove from heat and drain if there is anything remaining water. Place in a medium bowl.
    - In a medium pot, boil potatoes on high heat for 5 minutes (slightly longer for sweet potatoes). Drain and add to greens in bowl. Add ½ teaspoon salt and a sprinkle of black pepper. Add the apple cider vinegar.
    - Toast the pumpkin seeds in a skillet over low-medium heat, about 3-5 minutes, until fragrant and slightly browned. Stir into bowl with potatoes and greens.
    - Use a large casserole dish (13x9 or 10x15) to prepare the enchiladas. Coat the bottom of the dish with ½ cup enchilada sauce and a spoonful of the potato mixture. Warm the tortillas on a skillet over low heat, flipping them once (You may want to first lightly coat the skillet with coconut oil before heating them, so that they become soft rather than crispy).
    - Place the first tortilla in the baking pan and coat in the sauce on the bottom of the pan. Place ¼ cup of the potato filling on the tortilla and roll it. Repeat with the remaining tortillas and potato filling, adding more sauce as necessary to coat tortillas. Use another baking dish if you run out of space.
    - Cover the top of the enchiladas with the remainder of the filling. Add optional cheese on top. Bake for 20-25 minutes, covered with foil.

DESSERT

Tofu chocolate mousse

- Makes 6-8 servings
- Ingredients
    - 1 pound silken tofu
    - ½ cup medjool dates, soaked* and pitted (about 5 dates)
    - ½ cup maple syrup
    - 1 teaspoon vanilla extract
    - 1 bar (3.5oz) dark chocolate, at least 65% cacao, melted
    - 1 tablespoon cacao powder
    - ½ tablespoon cinnamon
- Instructions
    - Process dates and 1 tablespoon warm water in food processor until smooth. Add maple syrup, vanilla extract, and tofu and process to combine. Finally, add melted chocolate, cacao powder, and cinnamon and process until smooth and creamy.
    - Serve at room temperature or chilled.

[*To soak dates, cover in boiling water and allow to sit for 10 minutes before draining.]

Frozen banana soft serve

- Makes 4 servings
- Ingredients
    - 4 medium bananas, unpeeled and frozen
    - ½ teaspoon vanilla extract
    - 1-2 tablespoons plant-based milk such as unsweetened almond milk
    - Optional – 1 cup frozen cherries or strawberries (for cherry or strawberry-banana soft serve), ½ cup chocolate chips
- Instructions
    - Remove bananas from freezer and slice into 1-inch pieces.
    - In a food processor, process the frozen banana pieces and vanilla extract until creamy, adding plant-based milk if necessary.
    - If using cherries or strawberries, add and process until creamy. If using chocolate chips, add and pulse to combine.
    - Serve immediately.

Date and walnut bread

- Makes 8-10 slices
- Ingredients
    - 1 ½ cups medjool dates, soaked and pitted, chopped into small pieces
    - 2 cups boiling water
    - 1 ½ cups white whole wheat flour (you can also substitute with any amount of almond flour)
    - ½ cup oat flour (or rolled oats ground into flour)
    - 1 tablespoon baking soda
    - ½ tablespoon cinnamon
    - ¼ teaspoon salt
    - ½ cup honey
    - 1 teaspoon apple cider vinegar
    - ¾ cup plant-based milk such as unsweetened almond milk
    - ½ cup coconut oil, melted
    - 1 flax egg*, or 1 egg
    - ½ cup walnuts, chopped
- Instructions
    - Preheat oven to 350 degrees F. Coat a 9x5 baking pan in coconut oil or cooking spray.
    - In a medium bowl, whisk together the flour, baking soda, cinnamon, salt, and sugar.
    - In another bowl, whisk together the plant-based milk and vinegar until frothy. Add the coconut oil and egg or flax egg.
    - Add dry to wet ingredients and mix to combine. Add dates and walnuts. If mixture is too dry, add plant-based milk as needed.
    - Pour into baking pan and bake for 35-40 minutes

*Flax egg (vegan egg replacer)

-Mix 1 tablespoon ground flax meal with 3 tablespoons of warm water.
-Let sit for 5 minutes and allow to thicken.

Fudgy brownies

- ◊ Makes 12-16 brownies
- ◊ Ingredients
    - 1 ½ cups of semisweet chocolate chips, or 1 (3.5oz) bar of dark chocolate (65-72%), chopped
    - 1/3 cup coconut oil
    - 2/3 cup almond flour (You can substitute 1/3 cup with brown rice flour or garbanzo flour)
    - 2 tablespoons unsweetened cocoa powder
    - ½ teaspoon ground cinnamon
    - ½ teaspoon baking soda
    - ¼ teaspoon salt
    - 2 eggs
    - 1/3 cup maple syrup or honey
    - 1 teaspoon vanilla extract
    - ½ cup walnuts, chopped
- ◊ Instructions
    - Preheat the oven to 350°F. Lightly coat an 8x8 inch baking pan with coconut oil or cooking spray.
    - Melt 1 cup of chocolate chips or chopped dark chocolate over low heat in a saucepan. Add coconut oil, melt and whisk in to chocolate.
    - In a medium bowl, combine almond flour and, if using, brown rice or garbanzo flour. Mix in cocoa powder, cinnamon, baking soda, and salt.
    - In a large bowl, add eggs and whisk vigorously. Add maple syrup and honey and continue whisking. Add vanilla extract and melted chocolate. Whisk until smooth.
    - Add wet to dry ingredients and stir until just combined. Add remaining ½ cup chocolate chips or chunks and walnuts.
    - Pour mixture into prepared pan. Bake for 30 minutes, being careful not to overcook.
    - Let cool completely before cutting and serving.
    - Store in an airtight container in the refrigerator for up to 6 days or in the freezer for up to 3 months.

REFERENCES

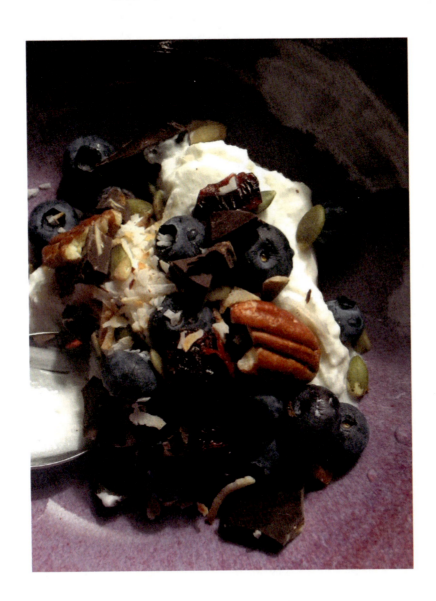

REFERENCES

GENERAL/INTRODUCTION

1. Katz D, Friedman R, Lucan S. Nutrition In Clinical Practice: A Comprehensive, Evidence-Based Manual for the Practitioner, 3rd ed. Philadelphia: Wolters Kluwer; 2015.
2. Schulte E, Avena N, Gearhardt A. Which Foods May Be Addictive? The Roles of Processing, Fat Content, and Glycemic Load. PLoS ONE 2015;10:1-18.
3. Iozzo P, Guiducci L, Guzzardi MA, Pagotto U. Brain PET Imaging in Obesity and Food Addiction: Current Evidence and Hypothesis. Obes Facts 2012;5:155-64.
4. Wang GJ, Volkow ND, et al. Brain dopamine and obesity. Lancet 357(9253);354-357.
5. Moore L, Thompson F. Adults Meeting Fruit and Vegetable Intake Recommendations – United States, 2013. Centers for Disease Control and Prevention Morbidity and Mortality Weekly Report 2015;64:709-13. Available at www.cdc.gov.
6. Esselstyn C, Gendy G, Doyle J, et al. A way to reverse CAD? J Fam Pract 2014;63:356-64.
7. Orlich MJ, Singh PN, Sabate J, et al. Vegetarian Dietary Patterns and Mortality in Adventist Health Study 2. JAMA 2013;173:1230-8.
8. Consumer Reports. Antibiotics are widely used by the US meat industry. Available at Consumerreports.org. Published 2012. Accessed October 7, 2016.
9. Gerber PJ, Steinfeld H, Henderson B, et al. Tackling climate change through livestock – A global assessment of emissions and mitigation opportunities. Food and Agriculture Organization of the United Nations (FAO). Published 2013.
10. Gerald J, Dorothy R. Are You Getting Enough Fiber? Tufts University Health & Nutrition Letter. Published 2016.
11. Katz D. The Paleo Diet: Can We Really Eat Like Our Ancestors Did? The Huffington Post. Published 2011. Available at huffingtonpost.com. Accessed April 6. 2017.
12. Huffington Post. Why You Should Never Peel an Apple. Huffington Post Healthy Living Published February 19, 2014. Available at huffingtonpost.com. Accessed April 16, 2017.

13. Wang D, Yanping Li, Chiuve S, et al. Association of Specific Dietary Fats with Total and Cause-Specific Mortality. JAMA 2016;176:1134-45.
14. Simopoulos A. Essential fatty acids in health and chronic disease. Am J Clin Nutr 1999;70(suppl):560S-9S.
15. Harvard Medical School. Glycemic index and glycemic load for 100+ foods: Measuring carbohydrate effects can help glucose management. Harvard Health Publications. Published August 27, 2015. Available at health.harvard.edu. Accessed April 16, 2017.
16. Johnston C, Kim C. Vinegar Improves Insulin Sensitivity to a High-Carbohydrate Meal in Subjects with Insulin Resistance or Type 2 Diabetes. Diabetes Care 2004;27:281-2.
17. Jarvill-Taylor K, Anderson R, Graves D. A hydroxychalcone derived from cinnamon functions as a mimetic for insulin in 3T3-L1 adipocytes. J Am Coll Nutr 2001;20:327-36.
18. Wolfe R, Cifelli A, Kostas G. Optimizing Protein Intake in Adults: Interpretation and Application of the Recommended Dietary Allowance Compared with the Acceptable Macronutrient Distribution Range. Advances in Nutrition 2017;8:266-75.
19. Institute of Medicine. Dietary Reference Intakes: RDA and AI for Total Water and Macronutrients. United States Department of Agriculture National Agricultural Library. Available at nal.usda.gov. Accessed April 21, 2017.
20. Pawlak R, Berger J, Hines I. Iron Status of Vegetarian Adults: A Review of the Literature. Am J Lifestyle Med 2016.
21. Institute of Medicine. Dietary reference intakes for vitamin A, vitamin K, arsenic, boron, chromium, copper, iodine, iron, manganese, molybdenum, nickel, silicon, vanadium, and zinc. Available at www.nap.edu. Accessed April 24, 2017.
22. Sundararaman S, Fonseca V, Alam M, Shah S. The Role of Iron in Diabetes and Its Complications. Diabetes Care 2007;30:1926-33.
23. Dohle S, Rall S, Siegrist M, et al. Does self-prepared food taste better? Effects of food preparation on liking. Health Psychology 2016;35:500-8.
24. Song K, Milner J. The Influence of Heating on the Anticancer Properties of Garlic. J Nutr 2001;131:1054S-57S.
25. Mullen W, Stewart A, Lean M, et al. Effect of freezing and storage on the phenolics, ellagitannins, flavonoids, and antioxidant capacity of red raspberries. J Agric Food Chem 2002;50:5197-201.

26. Harvard Medical School. Butter vs. Margarine. Harvard Health Publications Healthbeat. Available at health.harvard.edu. Accessed April 16, 2017.
27. McIndoo H. Breakfast Cereal Time. Environmental Nutrition 2016;5. Available at environmentalnutrition.com. Accessed October 13, 2016.
28. Boesler M. Bottled Water Costs 2000 Times As Much As Tap Water. Business Insider. Published July 12, 2013. Available at businessinsider.com. Accessed April 16, 2017.
29. Baranski M, Srednicka-Tober D, Volakakis N, et al. Higher antioxidant and cadmium concentrations and lower incidence of pesticide residues in organically grown crops: a systematic literature review and meta-analyses. Br J Nutr 2014;112:794-811.
30. Dangour A, Lock K, Hayter A. Nutrition-related health effects of organic foods: a systematic review. Am J Clin Nutr 2010;92:203-10.
31. National Cancer Institute. Agricultural Health Study. Published 2011. Available at cancer.gov. Accessed April 6, 2017.
32. Environmental Working Group. Dirty Dozen: EWG's 2016 Shopper's Guide to Pesticides in Produce. Available at ewg.org. Accessed October 20, 2016.
33. Bolton J, Bushway A, Crowe K, et al. Best Ways to Wash Fruits and Vegetables. University of Maine Cooperative Extension Publications. Published 2013. Available at extension.umaine.edu. Accessed March 2, 2016.
34. Zander A, Bunning M. Guide to Washing Fresh Produce. Colorado State University Extension 2010;3.
35. Elkins K. I compared the price of organic and regular items at Whole Foods – here's what I found. Business Insider. Published August 7, 2015. Available at businessinsider.com. Accessed April 16, 2017.
36. Consumer Reports. When it pays to buy organic. Consumer Reports 2006;71:12-17.
37. US Food & Drug Administration. Code of Federal Regulations Title 21, Part 101: Food Labeling. CFR 2016. Available at accessdata.fda.gov.
38. Givens D, Lovegrove J. Higher PUFA and n-3 PUFA, conjugated linoleic acid, alpha-tocopherol and iron, but lower iodine and selenium concentrations in organic milk: a systematic literature review and meta- and redundancy analyses. Br J Nutr 2016;116:1-2.
39. Weil A. Dr. Weil's Anti-Inflammatory Diet. Available at DrWeil.com. Accessed April 16, 2017.

40. Percival S, Vanden Huevel J, Nieves C, et al., Bioavailability of herbs and spices in humans as determined by ex vivo inflammatory suppression and DNA strand breaks. J Am Coll Nutr 2012;31:288-94.
41. Kamanger, F, Emadi, A. Vitamin and Mineral Supplements: Do We Really Need Them? Int J Prev Med 2012;3:221-26.
42. Kumar J, Muntner P, Kaskel FJ, et al. Prevalence and associations of 25-hydroxyvitamin D deficiency in US children: NHANES 2001-2004. Pediatr 2009;124:362-70.
43. Theodoratou E, Tzoulaki I, Zgaga L, Loannidis JPA. Vitamin D and multiple health outcomes: umbrella review of systematic reviews and meta-analyses of observational studies and randomized trials. BMJ 2014;348:g2035.
44. Ayers S, Baum A, McManus C, et al. Cambridge Handbook of Psychology, Health & Medicine; 2nd edition. Cambridge University Press, 2007.
45. Armstrong M, Mottershead T, Ronksley P, et al. Motivational interviewing to improve weight loss in overweight and/or obese patients: a systematic review and meta-analysis of randomized controlled trials. Obes Rev 2011;12:709-23.
46. University of Massachusetts. Motivational Interviewing Definition Principles Approach. Available at unmass.edu. Accessed April 6. 2017.
47. Gallagher M. USDA Defines Food Deserts. ANA Nutrition Digest 2011. American Nutrition Association. Available at americannutritionassociation.org. Accessed January 1, 2017.

OBESITY

48. Czernichow S, Kengne A, Stamatakis E, et al. Body mass index, waist circumference and waist-hip ratio: which is the better discriminator of cardiovascular disease mortality risk? Obes Rev 2011;12:680-7.
49. Harvard Medical School. The dubious practice of detox. Harvard Health Publications: Women's Health Watch May, 2008. Available at health.harvard.edu. Accessed April 16, 2017.
50. Mattson M, Longo V, Harvie M. Impact of Intermittent Fasting on Health and Disease Processes. Ageing Research Reviews 2016.

51. Gersema E. Fasting-like diet turns the immune system against cancer. USC News 2016. Available at news.usc.edu.
52. Ebbeling C, Feldman H, Osganian S, et al. Effects of Decreasing Sugar-Sweetened Beverage Consumption on Body Weight in Adolescents: A Randomized, Controlled Pilot Study. Pediatr 2016;117:673-80.
53. Larson N, Laska M, Story M, et al. Sports and energy drink consumption are linked to health-risk behaviours among young adults. Public Health Nutr 2014;18:2709-803.
54. McCarthy M. Soda tax brings sharp fall in sugary drink consumption in Californian city. BMJ 2016;355.
55. Tribole, E, Resch, E. Intuitive Eating, 3rd ed. New York: St. Martin's Griffin; 2012.
56. Mindfuleating.org. The S.T.O.P. Instructions. Mindfuleating.org: The CAMP System. DayOne Publishing 2010. Accessed December 12, 2016.
57. Reynolds G. The Limits of Intuitive Eating. The New York Times. Published Nov 2015. Available at well.blogs.nytimes.com. Accessed February 29, 2017.
58. Meier K. Foods and moods: Considering the future may help people make better food choices. ScienceDaily. Published February 12, 2014. Accessed March 12, 2017.

DIABETES

59. Pi-Sunyer F.X. How Effective Are Lifestyle Changes in the Prevention of Type 2 Diabetes Mellitus? Nutr Rev;65:101-9.
60. Knowler W, Barret-Connor E, Fowler S, et al. Reduction in the incidence of Type 2 Diabetes with lifestyle Intervention or Metformin. N Eng J Med 2002;346:393-403.
61. Chandalia M, Garg A, Lutjohann D, et al. Beneficial effects of high dietary fiber intake in patients with Type 2 Diabetes Mellitus. N Eng J Med 2000;342:1392-1398.
62. Shai I, Schwarzfuchs D, Yaakov H, et al. Weight Loss with a Low-Carbohydrate, Mediterranean, or Low-Fat Diet. N Eng J Med 2008;359:229-241.
63. Esposito K, Maiorino M, Petrizzo M, Bellastella G, Giugliano D. The Effects of a Mediterranean Diet on the Need for Diabetes Drugs and Remission of Newly Diagnosed Type 2 Diabetes: Follow-up of a Randomized Trial. Diabetes Care 2014;37:1824-30

64. Ley S, Hamdy O, Mohan V, et al. Prevention and Management of Type 2 Diabetes: Dietary Components and Nutritional Strategies. Lancet 2014;383:1999-2007.
65. National Cancer Institute. Artificial Sweeteners and Cancer. Available at cancer.gov. Accessed April 16, 2017.

CARDIOVASCULAR DISEASE

66. Centers for Disease Control and Prevention National Center for Health Statistics. Leading Causes of Death. March 17, 2017. Available at cdc.gov. Accessed April 16, 2017.
67. Ha V, de Souza R. "Fleshing Out" the Benefits of Adopting a Vegetarian Diet. J Am Heart Assoc 2015;4:1-3.
68. Hu F. Plant-based foods and prevention of cardiovascular disease: an overview. Am J Clin Nutr 2003;78(suppl):544S-51S.
69. Jenkins D, Kendall C, Marchie A, et al. Effects of a Dietary Portfolio of Cholesterol-Lowering Foods vs Lovastatin on Serum Lipids and C-Reactive Protein. JAMA 2003;290:502-510.
70. McDougall J, Thomas L, McDougall C, et al. Effects of 7 days on an ad libitum low-fat vegan diet: the McDougall Program cohort. Nutr J 2014;13.
71. Djousse L, Gaziano JM. Egg consumption in relation to cardiovascular disease and mortality: the Physicians' Health Study. Am J Clin Nutr. 2008; 84;964-9.
72. de Oliveira Otto M, Mozaffarian D, Kromhout D, et al. Dietary intake of saturated fat by food source and incident cardiovascular disease: the Multi-Ethnic Study of Atherosclerosis. Am J Clin Nutr 2012;96:397-404.
73. Vincent-Baudry S, Defoort C, Gerber M, et al. The Medi-RIVAGE study: reduction of cardiovascular disease risk factors after a 3-mo intervention with a Mediterranean-type diet or a low-fat diet. Am J Clin Nutr 2005;82:964-71.
74. Estruch R, Ros E, Salas-Salvado J, et al. Primary Prevention of Cardiovascular Disease with a Mediterranean Diet. N Eng J Med 2013;368:1279-90.
75. US Food and Drug Administration. The FDA takes step to remove artificial trans fats in processed foods. FDA 2015. Available at www.fda.gov.

76. Mejia S, Kendall C, Viguiliouk E, et al. Effect of tree nuts on metabolic syndrome criteria: a systematic review and meta-analysis of randomised controlled trails. BMJ Open 2014;4:1-16.
77. Greger, Michael. Which Nut Fights Cancer Better? Nutritionfacts.org 2014. Available at nutritionfacts.org. Accessed March 15, 2017.

HYPERTENSION

78. Appel LJ, Moore T, Obarzanek E, et al. A Clinical Trial of the Effects of Dietary Patterns on Blood Pressure. N Eng J Med 1997;336:1117-24.
79. Ostchega Y, Hughes J, Terry A, et al. Abdominal Obesity, Body Mass Index, and Hypertension in US Adults: NHANES 2007-2010. Am J Hypertens 2012;25:1271-8.
80. Steffan L, Kroenke C, Yu X, et al. Associations of plant food, dairy product, and meat intakes with 15-7 incidence of elevated blood pressure in young black and white adults: the Coronary Artery Risk Development in Young Adults (CARDIA) Study. Am J Clin Nutr 2005;82:1169-77.
81. He F, Li J, MacGregor G. Effect of longer term modest salt reduction on blood pressure: Cochrane systematic review and meta-analysis of randomised trials. BMJ 2013;346.
82. Chan Q, Stamler J, Elliot P. Dietary Factors and Higher Blood Pressure in African-Americans. Curr Hypertens Rep 2015;17
83. Centers for Disease Control. Alcohol and Public Health. Centers for Disease Control and Prevention 2016. Available at www.cdc.gov.

CANCER

84. Orlich M, Singh P, Sabate J, et al. Vegetarian dietary patterns and the risk of colorectal cancers. JAMA Intern Med 2015;175:767-76.
85. Harvard Health Publications. Cancer and diet: What's the connection? Harvard Health Publications: Harvard Men's Health Watch 2016.
86. Blot W, Tarone J. Doll and Peto's quantitative estimates of cancer risks: holding generally true for 35 years. J Natl Cancer Instit 2015;3:1-5.

87. Harvard Health Publications. Red meat and colon cancer. Harvard Health Publications: Harvard Men's Health Watch 2008.
88. Greger M. How Much Cancer Does Lunch Meat Cause? NutritionFacts.org. Published September 12, 2016. Accessed October 25, 2016.
89. Greger, M. Stool pH and Colon Cancer. NutritionFacts.org. Published February 23, 2015. Accessed October 25, 2016.
90. Holtan S, O'Connor H, Frederickson Z. Food-frequency questionnaire-based estimates of total antioxidant capacity and risk of Non-Hodgkin lymphoma. Int J Cancer 2012;131:1158-68.
91. Song W, Derito CM, Liu MK, et al. Cellular Antioxidant Activity of Common Vegetables. J Agric Food Chem 2010;58:6621-9.
92. Sun J, Chu Y, Wu X, et al. Antioxidant and Antiproliferative Activities of Common Fruits. J Agric Food Chem 2002;50:7449-54.

GASTROINTESTINAL DISEASE

93. The University of Chicago Medicine. Celiac Disease Facts and Figures. The University of Chicago Medicine Celiac Disease Center. Available at cureceliacdisease.org. Accessed April 16, 2017.
94. Biesiekierski, J, Peters S, Newnham E, et al. No Effects of Gluten in Patients With Self-Reported Non-Celiac Gluten Sensitivity After Dietary Reduction of Fermentable, Poorly Absorbed, Short-Chain Carbohydrates. Gastroenterology 2013;145:320-38.
95. Celiac.org. Sources of gluten. Celiac Disease Foundation 2017. Available at celiac.org. Accessed January 2, 2017.
96. IBS Diets. FODMAP Food List. IBSDiets.org 2016. Available at ibsdiets.org. Accessed January 4, 2017.
97. Goldsmith J, Sartor B. The role of diet on intestinal microbiota metabolism: Downstream impacts on host immune function and health, and therapeutic interventions. J Gastroenterol 2014;49:785-98.
98. Yoon J, Sohn W, Lee O, et al. Effect of multispecies probiotics on irritable bowel syndrome: A randomized, double-blind, placebo-controlled trial. J Gastroenterol Hepatol 2013;29:52-9.

99. Johnston B, Goldenberg J, Parkin P. Probiotics and the Prevention of Antibiotic-Associated Diarrhea in Infants and Children. JAMA 2016;316:1484-5.

NEUROLOGIC DISEASE

100. Victor M, Adams RA, Collins GH. The Wernicke-Korsakoff syndrome and related disorders due to alcoholism and malnutrition. FA Davis, Philadelphia 1989.
101. Parkin AJ, Blunden J, Rees JE, et al. Wernickee-Korsakoff syndrome of nonalcoholic origin. Brain Cognition 1991;15:69.
102. Martin V, Brinder V. Diet and Headache: Part 2. Headache Currents 2016;1553-62.
103. Mayo Clinic Staff. Caffeine content for coffee, tea, soda, and more. Mayo Clinic Nutrition and Healthy Eating 2014. Available online at mayoclinic.org. Accessed January 2, 2017.
104. Hardman R, Kennedy G, Macpherson H, et al. Adherence to a Mediterranean-Style Diet and Effects on Cognition in Adults: A Qualitative Evaluation and Systematic Review of Longitudinal and Prospective Trials. Frontiers in Nutrition 2016;3:22.
105. Horrocks L, Yeo Y. Health Benefits of Docosahexaenoic acid (DHA). Pharmacol Res 1999;40:211-25.
106. Cao L, Tan L, Wang H, et al. Dietary Patterns and Risk of Dementia: a Systematic Review and Meta-Analysis of Cohort Studies. Mol Neurobiol 2016;53:6144-54.

Made in the USA
Columbia, SC
23 June 2017